The Welcome Visitor
Living Well, Dying Well

JOHN HUMPHRYS

with

Dr Sarah Jarvis

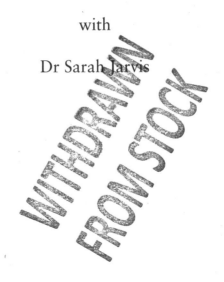

H
HODDER &
STOUGHTON

First published in Great Britain in 2009 by Hodder & Stoughton
An Hachette UK company

1

Copyright © John Humphrys and Sarah Jarvis 2009

The right of John Humphrys and Sarah Jarvis to be identified as
the Authors of the Work has been asserted by them in accordance
with the Copyright, Designs and Patents Act 1988.

A CIP catalogue record for this title is available from the British Library

Hardback ISBN 978 0340 923771
Trade paperback ISBN 9780340919279

Typeset in Sabon by Hewer Text UK Ltd, Edinburgh
Printed and bound by Clays Ltd, St Ives plc

Hodder & Stoughton policy is to use papers that are natural, renewable
and recyclable products and made from wood grown in sustainable
forests. The logging and manufacturing processes are expected to
conform to the environmental regulations of the country of origin.

Hodder & Stoughton Ltd
338 Euston Road
London NW1 3BH

www.hodder.co.uk

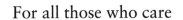

For all those who care

Contents

Acknowledgements

This book owes its existence to the thousands of people who wrote to me in 2003 after the death of my father. They told me about their own anguish and, often, sense of guilt over the unnecessary suffering of their own loved ones. I hope what follows helps reassure them that they are not alone. As always, my thanks to my longsuffering editors at Hodder: Rowena Webb, Helen Coyle and Cecilia Moore and to my equally longsuffering agent Luigi Bonomi. Dr Andrea Killick generously shared with me the fruits of her own research into death and dying in literature. Anne Naysmith, the palliative care consultant at Pembridge Hospice, gave Sarah invaluable help and guidance. Catherine Bennett gave me both uncritical encouragement and some sharply critical observations: the perfect combination. And Sarah proved that it is possible to work for years with the grumpiest of co-authors without resorting to physical violence. I am grateful to them all.

It is as natural to die as to be born
                                        Francis Bacon

Preface

It's a risky business, writing about something you've never experienced. The problem with death is that there is no other way to do it – on the basis that once you've actually experienced it, that's it. We don't get a practice run. We can't come back and talk about it and we don't get a second crack at it if it went badly the first time. On the other hand, there are plenty of people with tons of second-hand experience – doctors, nurses, hospice staff – who see it happening all the time. That's why the name of Dr Sarah Jarvis is on the cover of this book alongside my own. She has the knowledge that only a doctor who has practised as a GP for many years can have. Good doctors not only help keep people alive; they help them have a good death. But Sarah and I had a few differences to sort out before we could put pen to paper.

I have come to believe over the past few years – mostly because of the circumstances surrounding the death of my own father in 2003 – that there is a powerful case for some form of assisted suicide. Under certain, strictly regulated circumstances doctors should be allowed to help their patient die. By 'help', I mean more than just withholding treatment. That has always happened and the law allows it; I mean taking more active steps. Sarah was dubious. It flew in the face of everything she had been trained to do as a doctor and, more importantly, what she personally believed was ethically and morally acceptable.

In the years following my father's death Sarah and I agreed that we had been arguing about the wrong thing. This is not about a cold, clinical procedure in which a doctor stands at the bedside of a sick person and calmly administers the injection that will stop the heart beating. This is about recognising that there is such a thing as a life force or, if you prefer, the will to live, and what should happen when that disappears. There should be a recognition that, just as we expect to have control over our own lives, so we should have control over our own deaths.

Ask doctors or nurses to define the life force and they cannot, any more than an astro-physicist can define the dark matter that makes up most of the universe. But they know it is there. They have seen it in the chaotic A and E department of a district hospital when the victims of an accident are being brought in; on a cancer ward for the terminally ill; in the hush of an intensive care unit where a patient fights for life. And they have heard it in the howling cacophony of a maternity hospital where new life is coming into being.

They know when it is present and they know

when it begins to fade. And so do those of us who have no medical knowledge or experience but who have witnessed a life nearing its end. It may be the cancer sufferer who has finally surrendered to the inevitable, or it may even be the husband or wife who has died within weeks of their partner even though there was very little clinically wrong with them. They simply lost the will to live.

As every life is unique, so is every death. I have been with three people – each of whom was very close to me for many years – in the final hours of their lives, and each time it was very different. My brother died suddenly. It happened in a matter of weeks following a diagnosis of cancer. My former wife had many months to prepare for what she knew was inevitable. My father had wanted to die for many years. In his case the will to live disappeared with the death of my mother. And yet he was treated – if that's the right word – as though he embraced life and treasured every extra day. That cannot be right. GPs like Sarah see this all the time. The policy of her professional organisation, the British Medical Association (BMA), is to oppose any form of assisted suicide. She now believes that is wrong. So do most other people in this country – at least according to the opinion polls. They want society to think again about how we deal with people for whom life has lost all meaning. That's one of the reasons for writing this book.

When I first thought about doing so in 2003

Sarah and I gave very little thought to whether the laws should be changed to allow doctors to help people die. Since then the debate has taken off, not only in Britain but in other countries too, and the pressure for change seems to be acquiring an unstoppable momentum. As I write, the voters of Washington State in the USA have voted for just such a change in the law. This side of the Atlantic in tiny Luxembourg it has taken a bizarre twist. The monarch, Grand Duke Henri, has been stripped of his political powers because he tried to veto a bill that would allow assisted suicide.

But there is another, equally important reason for this book and that is to address the question of what we mean by a good death. Two thousand years ago the philosopher Seneca wrote, 'He will live badly who does not know how to die well.' But what do we mean today by 'dying well' and, even if we know what we want for ourselves, how can we apply that to a loved one who relies on us in the final stages of life? Ancient philosophers aren't much help here, and nor is the modern medical profession. The extraordinary advances in palliative care over the past few decades and the armoury of drugs in every pharmacy mean few people should die in pain these days, but there is much more to a good death than freedom from pain at the end. And anyway, even with the best that modern palliative medicine has to offer, it is not possible to guarantee everyone a death without pain or severe discomfort. What is possible is to prepare ourselves, both philosophically and practically, for our own death and the deaths of our loved ones. There is a great deal that can be done, and this book offers both some observations and, we hope, some useful guidance.

We in the developed world have a problem that our ancestors did not face. We tend to live much longer. Death is now more often a gradual process rather than a sudden, cataclysmic event. Where our grandparents might have seen it as a candle being instantly snuffed out, we are much more likely to see it as the light slowly fading. In many ways that is a comforting thought, but the danger is that the extra years will prove more curse than blessing. The eternal wish is for a long life and a happy one. Sadly, the one does not necessarily follow from the other.

The biggest fear for most of us is dementia, the disease that has been most graphically described as dying from the inside out and which is so disgracefully neglected when research funds are handed out. The number of people with Alzheimer's and other brain diseases is growing at a frightening rate quite simply because we are living for so much longer. They suffer more than we can know because we cannot enter what remains of their minds. But they are not the only victims. Their relatives and friends suffer too. Millions of lives in this country alone are touched – often destroyed – by the horror of watching someone descending into the depths of dementia, losing everything that made them the people we loved.

Many of those who sacrifice everything to care for them must do so alone. They have to face the greatest challenge imaginable without the emotional support of the person they once shared their lives with: the person who might have been their lover, their best friend, their helpmate, their confidante. In the relentlessly destructive world of Alzheimer's, the once-loved husband, wife or parent often becomes a stranger – sometimes hostile and endlessly demanding, sometimes sunk into a misery so deep that it is impossible to penetrate it and make any contact.

We make light of our fading faculties when it is safe to do so: all those jokes that seem so inconsequential in our middle age when we can't remember why we've gone upstairs or the name of the book we are enjoying so much or even the name of our partner as we try to introduce them at a party. It's mildly embarrassing at the time but worth a chuckle later. The humour fades pretty quickly when we are faced with the reality of dementia.

My own sister was stricken with Alzheimer's in her early sixties and for a while we all joined in her amusement at her silly little memory lapses. By the time we realised they weren't so silly, she was no longer able to understand what was happening to her. She didn't even remember that she had been diagnosed with cancer a year or so earlier. Maybe God does have a sense of humour after all.

Those who have to care for people with dementia cannot expect gratitude or even recognition for their efforts and many end up hoping and praying that death will come to the victim sooner rather than later. The guilt they feel for wishing their loved one dead can be at best corrosive and at worst destructive. I hope this book succeeds in helping those who experience that guilt to realise that they are not alone, and that it is the most natural thing in the world to want to see an end to their loved one's suffering. If it helps persuade even a few movers and shakers to take Alzheimer's much more seriously, that's good too. When the begging bowl is extended it may not have the public appeal and high profile of cancer, but it is every bit as worthy.

So Sarah and I wrote this book for the same reasons but from two different perspectives. Incidentally, Sarah's sections are marked with the symbol of a doctor's bag to distinguish them from my own. Sarah has to deal on an almost daily basis with the consequences of her own professional achievements: helping people to live longer. I have nothing like her experience but, in common with so many others, I have seen the slow death from dementia of people close to me and wondered why they had to suffer as they did. The picture of a desperate daughter trying to cope with a demented mother at the same time as she is trying to raise her own family is something from which we would prefer to avert our gaze – partly because we simply do not know how to help, but mostly because we fear something similar may happen to us one day.

There is nothing glamorous or heroic about this battle, and there are no miracle cures on the horizon. Yet we can accept that death is inevitable without also meekly accepting that the closing years hold nothing but fear, despair and loss of dignity. What this book sets out to say is that it does not have to be like that.

At last society is beginning to accept that we should have some control over our own fate when our body or mind begins to fail. But that's all it is: a beginning. Sarah and I will argue that society's approach to death must change as we all live longer. We want to suggest ways in which things might be better. These are perhaps the most profound and troubling issues facing the Western world. By failing to confront them we condemn millions to unnecessary suffering.

If I had any doubts about the extent of public disquiet on this subject they were dispelled when my own programme, *Today*, broadcast a series of reports on it in the summer of 2008. We had a huge number of calls, letters and emails from people who said, in effect, that they were afraid of living too long and might end up having no control over how their lives ended.

Some years ago I heard one of the few survivors of the Auschwitz concentration camp talking about how he and his fellow victims had tried to cope in that terrible place. One of them had been a musician, who found some solace in composing small pieces of music on scraps of paper. He had no illusions as to his fate, and death held no fear for him given the horror of his life. The name he gave one of his pieces was the inspiration for the title of this book. I hope our book will do something to relieve the guilt of those who secretly regard death as a welcome visitor but are afraid to say so.

Death is not the greatest of evils; it is worse to want to die, and not be able to.

Sophocles

I

A Sense of Guilt and Betrayal

The sun was just beginning to edge above the horizon as I drove across the Severn Bridge. At the legal speed limit it takes less than a minute to cross from Wales into England, but I drove slowly. I wanted that minute to stretch. That was partly because of the beauty of the dawn. The sun's early rays flashed through the gaps between the cables supporting the roadway and glinted off the wide waters of the estuary. There is something special about crossing a suspension bridge – the sense of being almost airborne and the surprise that this seemingly delicate, spider-web structure can support such a massive weight. But it was also because I had left part of my life in Wales.

Ahead of me in London was a party to celebrate my sixtieth birthday. Of all our birthdays, the sixtieth is the least ambiguous. At forty we are still young. At fifty we are into comfortable middle age. By sixty we are beginning the final movement in the symphony of our lives. However long it may last, we can no longer pretend to youth.

For my father the symphony had reached its sombre climax a few hours earlier. He had died in the small hours of the morning. By a curious symmetry it happened in a modern unit built on the site of an old hospital in Cardiff where one of his grandchildren – my elder son Christopher – had been born thirty-seven years earlier. Death so often arrives in the small hours, that cold and cruel time when body and soul are at their weakest and, statistically, we are most likely to give up. Every nurse in every hospice and hospital in the land knows it.

I had dreaded the return to London – alone in the car for two or three hours, emotionally drained and physically exhausted. The penalty of presenting a programme like *Today* is that your sleep balance is permanently running an overdraft. When you need to draw on the account to help you through a sleepless night there is nothing there. As I left them, my family in Cardiff had worried that I might fall asleep at the wheel. They had no need to worry. It was a glorious dawn that held the promise of a perfect midsummer's day. I lowered all the windows and, for a few miles, let the warm wind buffet me. Far from dozing off, I was invigorated – even exhilarated. But surely this was wrong? Surely I should have been consumed with sorrow and sad memories, struggling to see the motorway through tears of grief?

When I had set out from my home in London twenty-four hours earlier to see my father alive for the last time I had intended to cancel the party. Yet now I was looking forward to it. How could this be? How could I be so callous? Should I, at the very least, be feeling guilt instead of anticipating the company of friends?

Perhaps I should have felt all that, but that's not how it was. Instead, when we stood in my garden a few hours later and drank a toast to the memory of my father, it felt like a moment of celebration rather than sorrow. The truth is – shocking as it may look in cold print – that I was glad he had died. So were my sister and brothers and his grandchildren and all those who knew and loved him. He had wanted to die for a very long time. For the first time in several years we were able to feel that he was truly at peace. Why should we feel guilt at the end of suffering? Why should death not be a welcome visitor? The blindingly obvious answer to that question is that it depends on the circumstances.

In my half-century as a journalist I have seen a great deal of death and disaster: floods and famines; earthquakes and wars. Nothing had made a more powerful impact on me than what happened at Aberfan in 1966, when a massive coal tip slid on to the primary school and crushed it like a boulder flattening a matchbox. It was a foul mix of mud and slurry, and it had raced down the hillside at terrible speed. The miners working on the surface at the village colliery heard its roar and delivered the awful news to the men deep below ground as they worked at the face. They raced to the surface and were there when I arrived in the village. Their faces were still black with coal dust, white streaks made by sweat and tears coursing down their cheeks as they dug for the bodies of their own children. One hundred and sixteen children died, and twenty-eight adults. I have been back to Aberfan many times since that awful day and the grief is still raw. It could hardly be otherwise. Those children had been cheated of life.

My sister died when I was a small boy. My mother's hair went white almost literally overnight and she grieved for her lost baby until her own death nearly half a century later. A parent never fully recovers from the death of a child. It is not the natural order of things.

But why does our culture find it so difficult to accept that death in old age is a part of life and is often to be welcomed? Why must we rage against the dying of the light even when the light has long since vanished from the eyes of those we love?

There were many reasons to celebrate my father's life. It was a long one – he was ninety-one – and often a hard one. He was once so poor he had to pawn my mother's engagement ring. But it had been a good life.

He was born into a working-class family in what I suppose we would now call a slum: a tiny inner-city house with an outdoor lavatory and a tin bath in front of the fire. He got measles when he was twelve. On a bright winter's day, when the sun glinted off the snow and his mother was out of the house, he ignored her warnings, left his darkened bedroom and slipped out into the glaringly white street. He paid for that act of childish disobedience with his eyesight.

His blindness lasted for a few years and that was the end of his education. Although his sight came back it never did so properly. But he was a tough character. He became a fine french polisher. He used my mother's eyes to tell him if he had managed to achieve a perfect colour match. If she voiced the slightest doubt – a bit too red, perhaps? – he would return to his shelves of bottles and tins, each full of different dyes and stains, powders and liquids, until he found exactly the right mix. He was one of the last of the old school of french polishers. After sixty years doing it, he told me he was still learning his trade. He was once talked into buying a spray gun, which would have made his life a lot easier but it lasted only a few days and ended up in the bin.

He was a good athlete, too – inordinately proud of having run for his county. He could have been even better, but it's not easy to race if you cannot see the man in front of you clearly. Once he ran off the course and into a barbed wire fence. He kept going. He always did.

Only when my mother died in 1990 did he give up. He turned to drink and downed at least a bottle of whisky a day until the inevitable happened and he collapsed. That was when he should have been allowed to die. He had, as he saw it, nothing left to live for.

He could no longer do any of the things he loved – not least his gardening and his long walks – and he missed my mother dreadfully. But far, far worse, he had stopped being the man he once was. His personality had changed.

Always difficult and argumentative, he had a deep distrust of all forms of authority. He once walked out of his crowded Conservative club rather than sit in the only vacant seat – which happened to be beneath a portrait of the Queen. You did not get many Tory republicans in working-class Cardiff. If a servant ever tried to send him to the tradesmen's entrance when he arrived at the front door of a posh house to polish the grand piano, he would turn on his heel and walk away. As he saw it, he was a skilled craftsman running his own one-man business – not that he was very good at the business side of things. He tended to charge people what he thought they could afford. The only reason for his being self-employed was that he had punched his foreman on the nose for some real or (probably) imagined slight when he had only just finished his apprenticeship, and got the sack. In those days jobs were not easy to come by. Of one thing he was certain: he was the equal of any man, whatever his wealth, status or so-called breeding.

In the closing years of his life he became vindictive, even vicious. He would turn on his children, especially my sister, who showed him more love and care than a parent had any right to expect, and lacerate her with his tongue. He seemed to take pleasure from inflicting pain. Because he was a clever man he was very good at it and we were growing to hate him for it. Much too late we came to realise what was happening. He was ill. Dementia was setting in. It was no more his fault that his personality was changing than it is the fault of a child who gets leukaemia.

We tried to make allowances and to get him treatment. We secretly arranged for a psychiatrist to see him at his home so we could find out more about what was happening to him. But he did not want a psychiatrist, spotted the ruse almost immediately and, when she arrived under some pretext or other, sent her packing. He did not want help. In his own eyes he did not need it. He wanted no treatment that would compromise his powerful sense of his own dignity and independence. What he really wanted was to die. He said so endlessly and I believe he meant it. The whisky was his suicide pill.

Eventually, it almost worked. When he collapsed, he was taken into a general hospital and hovered on the brink of death. He was treated as though he had had an awful accident and everything must be done to save him. We talked to the doctor on his ward and did our best to explain things to him, but you cannot tell a doctor to let your father die. Or so I thought. The drips and the drugs and the care did their work and he recovered – after a fashion.

The next year was hell. It was clear he could never return to his own home nor come to live in ours, because he needed constant care. He stayed for months in hospital, occupying a bed needed by people who were acutely ill. Eventually we found a private nursing home prepared to take him – but not for long. He was too disturbed to benefit from the care they could offer and they could not cope with his erratic and occasionally violent behaviour.

He was transferred to what had been a Victorian mental hospital and still looked and felt like one. He was in a pitiful state. For hours on end he would shout, 'Help! Help!' until his voice grew hoarse. I have no doubt in the slightest that he was shouting for an end to his miserable existence. The medical staff struggled to find the right balance of drugs to 'stabilise' his condition, but never quite succeeded.

Then a new EMI hospital (elderly mentally infirm) was opened in Cardiff and he was taken there. It was light years from the wretched, tiled corridors of the old mental institution: bright and breezy and with a staff who could not have shown more love and care if he had been their own father. Unlike us, his children who had been so hurt by the man he had become, they were immediately able to see behind the illness to the man he had once been. But still – for all the hugs from the lovely Josie and other staff – his life was utterly meaningless. There was the odd lucid moment when his memory returned with fierce accuracy to his young days, but mostly he dozed in a chair, grew weaker and longed for death.

Inevitably the day came when he decided to give up altogether. He stopped eating and drinking and death seemed close. We had been here before and he had been brought back from the brink by the paraphernalia of modern medicine. But this time it was different.

I sat in the sunlit waiting room with the doctor in charge of him and we talked not of life, but of death. He took me aback by quoting from the Victorian poet Arthur Hugh Clough. They were words that, I believe, should be inscribed on the wall of every doctor in the land who might one day have to deal with someone like my father: 'Thou shalt not kill; but need'st not strive officiously to keep alive.'

The consultant trotted out all the clinical jargon about the consequences of failing to treat him and withholding antibiotics; about the effects of severe dehydration and the various steps that could be taken to deal with it. But when I asked, 'What would we be keeping him alive for?' he paused and nodded, understanding perfectly what lay behind my question. He abandoned the language of science and used a phrase that you do not need to be a doctor to understand. He said simply and unemotionally, 'He has turned his face to the wall.'

In the end it was tacitly agreed that nature should be allowed to take its course. If he were in pain or discomfort, then of course he would be treated accordingly. Otherwise he would be allowed to die. And so it happened.

His last few hours were, I think, relatively peaceful, with his family at his bedside and enough morphine to ease his restlessness and perhaps hasten the end. His last few years had been anything but peaceful. He should not have suffered as he did. There was never the slightest hope that he would recover and lead anything like a happy, fulfilling life. Dementia does not work like that.

In some ways, as I have suggested, my father's death is the reason for this book. Or perhaps it would be more accurate to say that his life is the reason. He did nothing exceptional, nothing to earn him even the briefest mention in the history books. He was a decent, honest man who did the best he could with the talent and the opportunity that fate bequeathed him. He seldom complained; he just got on with it. In other words, he was no different from countless millions of others. But, like millions of others, he was betrayed at the end of his life.

He was entitled to spend his closing years in the dignity he so valued. He was stripped of that dignity when he lost his rational powers, because society simply does not know how to deal with the man he became. It's true that there are many in the health service and in hospices around the country who do their best to care for people like him but, through no fault of their own, their best is seldom good enough. And he was one of the lucky ones. I shudder at the thought of him having to stay in that ghastly old mental hospital or – much worse – one of the few really bad homes where the inmates (I choose that word with precision) are treated with contempt by the people who are meant to care for them.

We are all shamed by the stories that occasionally emerge of old people kept in a permanent zombie-like state, strapped into chairs, sometimes slowly starving to death because the staff cannot be bothered to make sure they eat something. We would not allow it to happen to children – there would be a national uproar – but when it's old people we make a few disapproving noises, shudder inwardly and get on with our lives. Perhaps we do not want to dwell on it too much because we fear that it may well happen to us one day. The awful truth is that we simply do not know how to deal with senility. It is a merciless enemy and we have no defence against it – nor even a strategy that might one day provide one.

My father's last years cast a shadow over what had been a good life, and those of us who knew and loved him feel a mixture of resentment and guilt to this day. We also face a long list of questions prompted by that guilt. These are a few of them:

- Did we do everything we could to give him the help he needed when it became clear that he was suffering from some form of dementia?
- Could we, in those bleak hours when he shouted himself hoarse at the wretchedness of his existence, have done more to rescue him from it?
- Should we, in one way or another, have helped him end it?
- If so ... how?
- And if it meant breaking the law, would we have been strong enough, determined enough, to face the consequences?

Many of us have shared the agony of those wretched defendants who appear from time to time in the docks of our criminal courts charged with putting an end to the life of the person they loved. I suspect most of us have silently applauded when a compassionate judge has allowed them to go free. What possible purpose could be served by adding to their punishment? They were, after all, acting out of love rather than hate, out of mercy rather than malice. And yet the law says they were guilty of a serious crime.

In the course of researching this book I have heard many people say: 'If I'd had the needle I'd have stuck it in his arm – whatever the law may say.' But would they? And can it be right that they should have even had to contemplate that awful deed?

Before we address those profoundly difficult questions, let's look at how we got to where we are today. That, at least, is simple enough: it's because we live so much longer than our forebears.

It seemed to him a cruel and unjust trick that fate had played upon him. He could have understood it if he had led a wild life, if he had drunk too much, played around with women or kept late hours. But he had done none of these things. It was monstrously unfair.

Mr Chester in Somerset
Maugham's *Sanatorium*

2

The Monster of Old Age

My father's life spanned two distinct periods in our social history. His own father could expect life to be nasty, brutish and short. We, his children, born in the mid-twentieth century, could expect the opposite. We were destined for an easy time of it – perhaps the easiest of any generation there has ever been and (assuming the scientists are right about global warming) the easiest there will ever be.

The blessings are easy to count: the continent of Europe more or less at peace; an end to the military conscription which sent so many of our young men off to die in vast numbers on foreign battlefields; an unimaginable growth in prosperity; the greatest improvements in education and physical wellbeing of any period in history.

No longer would under-nourished children, their thin bones weakened by rickets, be a common sight on the streets of our cities. Poverty would be defined in terms that would astonish an earlier generation. From now on children would be deemed poor if there were no foreign holidays or if bedrooms had to be shared after a certain age. In other words, luxuries that would have been unimaginable a few generations ago had become commonplace.

And as we grew richer, so we grew healthier. Vaccinations and antibiotics did for our generation what clean water and decent sanitation had done for the Victorians. When I was a timid four-year-old and my friends and I took our first nervous steps into the classroom of our infants' school we expected to see at least a handful of other little tots clumping around in clumsy metal leg braces, crippled by polio. By the time I had made it to grammar school that hideous disease had been defeated by the tiny drop of vaccine on the sugar lump we were given to suck as we stood shivering in our vests in the under-heated school gym. The disease that had almost carried me off when I was a small baby was the ubiquitous whooping cough and that, too, was in its final murderous phase by the time I left infants' school. So were the other big child-killers, especially diphtheria. Soon even tuberculosis and smallpox would become little more than the stuff of nightmares.

It's not that life was easy in the immediate post-war years for the vast majority of the population who made up the working class. On the contrary: anyone who paints a rose-coloured view of the fifties could not have lived through those years of numbing austerity. But by the sixties things were getting better, and they kept getting better.

Compared with my grandparents' lives things were less nasty in almost every sense, less brutish, and we could expect to live much, much longer.

What this did not mean, of course, was that we became content with our lot. The world does not work like that. We found new things to worry about instead – the sort of things that would have baffled my parents and their generation. Hard-pressed mothers today may worry about being able to afford the latest trainers or designer gear to save their children from the ridicule of their peers, but my parents and their friends had no such worries: every scruffy little kid in the neighbourhood had one set of clothes, which we wore to school and everywhere else, and possibly a cheap suit for Sunday best. When the shoes (black leather lace-ups) wore out, they either went to the cobbler's or were mended at home on iron lasts. When we grew out of them the money was somehow found to buy another pair. I never remember having more than one pair of shoes. In summer we wore what we called 'daps' – cheap white canvas shoes (plimsolls in the language of posh kids) which were daubed with Blanco when they got dirty. My parents did not have to worry about cars because nobody in the street had one – any more than they had indoor lavatories or any of the other little luxuries. As my mother often put it: what you've never had and never see, you never miss.

What changed our approach to the material world more than anything was commercial television. The advertisements took us into middle-class homes that were different from our own and they delivered a simple message: this is how the other half lives, so why not you? The obvious answer was that we could not afford to, but then hire purchase arrived – though not in my house because my parents regarded borrowing as a sin – and the age of consumerism came with it.

Throughout history the big challenge for the vast majority of the working class had been how to earn enough to keep body and soul together: how to fill stomachs and keep a roof over our heads. Then, in the space of a generation, we became 'consumers'. The new prosperity meant that even people who were relatively poor started buying what they wanted instead of what they needed. But even that huge change was modest compared with the revolution brought about by health improvements.

Longevity changed our attitudes to death just as consumerism changed our attitude to life. Now we have a new set of worries. Let's imagine the concerns of a working-class couple born in the late nineteenth century with another born a few decades ago. They are fictitious in name only: their experiences were common to their time.

Albert worked in a factory in one of the big northern cities and his wife Ethel cared for their growing family. Their roles were distinct: he earned the money and she spent it – very, very carefully. The smallest unexpected incident – Albert breaking his arm at work, as he once did – would throw the family finances into chaos. With so many small children, medical bills were a huge drain on resources too. The children were often sick. Their parents had lost one baby when Ethel was giving birth and they lost another to polio when he was four or five. The little boy breathed his final, gasping breaths in an iron lung.

Albert, too, was having difficulty breathing. He had also been coughing up blood – only small amounts, but he knew what it meant. It was a death sentence. Even if he had been able to afford the medical bills and the cost of a decent sanatorium, it was unlikely that he would live much beyond his late forties. Not that there was anything particularly unusual about that. Few working-class people born in the nineteenth century could expect to pass fifty. Death was almost always present one way or another in the tiny, cramped rooms of a big city slum. It was a rare month when the blinds were not drawn in one of the houses in the neighbourhood and a coffin laid out in the tiny front parlour.

Albert was desperately worried about how Ethel would cope after he passed away. The oldest boy was now twelve and beginning to bring in a little cash, but Albert could not see how she would manage to pay the rent, feed and clothe the children and meet all the other bills when she was a widow. On one level he felt he'd had a reasonable life – neither better nor worse than most of his contemporaries – but when he got on his knees at night he prayed for a few extra years and the chance to earn enough money to save Ethel and the children from the workhouse.

Three generations later Charlie and Lizzie, who had had children pretty late in life and were spending a small fortune on their education, thought a lot about longevity too – but for precisely the opposite reason from Albert. They would never admit it to anyone else, of course, but their worry was that their parents were living too long. They were in their late eighties and making increasing demands on their children – demands they were not at all sure they would be able to meet. Charlie's mother and Lizzie's father were both clearly becoming senile and could not live at home for very much longer. But their savings had been used up (they had thought they were pretty

*well off when they retired all those years ago,
and spent accordingly) and the care homes
would have to be paid for by their children.
That wasn't going to be easy. Nor was it easy
coping with parents who were slowly becoming
different people.*

*The easy-going relationship they had all
enjoyed when Charlie and Lizzie married
had turned into something horribly different.
Charlie's mother – a friendly, funny woman
who loved her grandchildren – was becoming
increasingly unpleasant, even with the youngest
child. It was painful watching it happen, but
what could they do? Everyone knew what was
going on, but no one – least of all her husband
– was prepared to raise it with her. Did she
know? Did she realise she was suffering from
the early stages of some sort of dementia?
Quite possibly, and that might explain her
dreadful mood swings. But it did not make
things any easier.*

*What was certain was that both the elderly
parents would have to go into a home before
long – there was no question of them moving
in with Charlie and Lizzie and their children
– and the cost would be enormous. Charlie's
mother had always joked that when she started
going barmy she wanted to be 'put down'. 'I
don't want to end up as one of those poor,*

*sad souls strapped to their chairs in a roomful
of other senile old biddies, watching telly all
day and waiting to die,' she used to say. 'I
want to go when I'm ready and with all my
faculties still working.' Was it just a joke, or
did she really mean it? What if she became
physically ill? How much of an effort should be
made to treat her, given the inevitable course
of her dementia? They were hellishly difficult
questions, and they would become more
pressing with every passing year.*

*There were times when Charlie almost
wished that the breast cancer his mother had
fought off a few years ago had ended her
life. At least she would have been spared this
suffering and – if he were to be entirely honest
with himself – his family would have been
spared the terrible anguish and upheaval that
the coming years would bring. He knew it was
wrong to think such a thing and he was deeply
ashamed of it, but he couldn't help himself.*

As I write today there are more than seven hundred
thousand people in Britain alone with some form
of dementia. When I first wrote about my father's
death in 2003 I was overwhelmed with letters from
people like the fictional Charlie and Lizzie. In each
case, their suffering touched the lives of several
other people – their wife or husband or sibling, and

probably one or more of their children too. So it is safe to say that the lives of millions of people are being affected by this single disease. This is not just a problem: it amounts to a crisis in the Western world and it is one that we have more or less chosen to ignore.

The amount of money spent on trying to find a cure for Alzheimer's in the United Kingdom is less than a pound per person per annum and the help given to those who must care for its victims often falls far below what they are entitled to expect and what they deserve. Compare this picture with the efforts being made to find cures or effective treatments for cancer or various forms of heart disease. I am not suggesting for a moment that they are not worthy causes. What I am saying is that dementia is every bit as worthy. Yet we do not see famous pop stars and Hollywood idols wearing little ribbons to declare their support for research into dementia. We do not have special days set aside in the calendar to draw our attention to the cause and seek support for it. It is simply not fashionable.

As a journalist for more than half a century I cannot pretend that this surprises me. A deranged old man making a terrible nuisance of himself does not have the heart-tugging appeal of a little boy with leukaemia or a beautiful pop diva with breast cancer. But the cost of this crisis in Britain alone is staggering. It was estimated at about £15 billion in 2007 – more than the combined cost of dealing with cancer, heart disease and strokes in that year. The reason politicians do not get more exercised about this huge outlay is that so much of it is accounted for by social care – a vast amount of which never makes it on to the accounting ledger. There is an army of unpaid carers – friends and relatives – who labour night and day for no financial reward. They do it out of a sense of responsibility or out of love. Without them the cost would simply be unsustainable. In some ways, they are the biggest victims of all.

So it is not only heartless to ignore the crisis of dementia, it is foolish. Our own selfish interest demands that we take it far more seriously than we have been doing. The number of people in the Western world with dementia is increasing sharply year by year. Within a generation it will have passed one million just in Britain. In the United States it has been calculated that 46 per cent of people over the age of eighty-five have some form of dementia. If we reach the age of eighty there is a one-in-five risk that we will develop it. Imagine boarding a plane, knowing there is a 20 per cent risk of it crashing before it reaches its destination. You'd find another way of getting there, wouldn't you? And the reason we can be certain that there will be more dementia is that we are living so much longer. I almost wrote 'too long', but how long is too long? Clearly that depends on what old age does to us.

A century ago the average life expectancy was forty-five for men and forty-nine for women. Of every four children born, one died before their first birthday. After childhood the big killers were lung problems. Tuberculosis (or consumption as they called it) was the worst. Next came pneumonia. Working-class people such as Albert, who could not escape the foul air of their factories or the smog of the big cities, were especially vulnerable. He and Ethel would simply not have understood the concept of living too long.

There are many people today who think they are ancient when they hit fifty and behave as though they are ninety. There are also people who have reached a hundred and behave as though they are fifty – often with their sense of humour intact. A very old French woman, Jeanne Calmant, was asked if she worried about looking old and said, 'No. I've only ever had one wrinkle, and I'm sitting on it.' It might not have been the funniest joke of all time, but it wasn't bad for someone who was celebrating her 110th birthday. She died in 1977 at the age of 122 – officially the oldest person in the world.

The great American comedian George Burns, who also notched up his century, kept his wits sharp to the end too. He said, 'If you live to be a hundred you've got it made. Very few people die past that age.'

That really was a good joke, but it was based on what has turned out to be a hugely mistaken assumption. For the past century or so the average lifespan has been increasing at the rate of two years for every decade. By the middle of the twentieth century 60 per cent of the population were still alive in their mid-sixties. Today, men can expect to live to seventy-five and women about six years longer. Charlie and Lizzie's children can reasonably expect to add a decade to that. In 2008 the Office of National Statistics published figures which showed that two-thirds of boys and three-quarters of girls born in 2001 will reach the age of eighty-five. And one in three of today's primary school children will live to be a hundred.

But although we have been remarkably successful at delaying death, we have not been so good at delaying ageing. Where death used to be something that struck suddenly – usually as the result of an infection of some sort – it now comes mostly after a long overture. The 'wasting disease' the Victorians so dreaded because it would have finished them off within months, if not weeks, is now identified as, say, a form of cancer that can be fought and often defeated. Nowadays after a run-in with such an illness we are still alive years later – alive to die of something else. The implications of all this are enormous for every one of us as individuals and for society as a whole.

The Victorian snake oil salesman in a checked suit and spats promising immortality to anyone daft enough to hand over sixpence for his bottle of coloured water may cut a ludicrous figure to us today, but now we come under a different kind of pressure from a different kind of huckster. The new sales pitch is more subtle and more seductive. It doesn't quite say, 'Great news! We really can live for ever!', but it does encourage the notion that we may well be able to stave off death indefinitely.

When I look in the mirror in the morning I see a man of sixty-five. This surprises me. Am I really that old? I doubt that it surprises anyone else. My face has all the lines and wrinkles you might expect of a man born when Britain was still at war with Germany – and then some. Kind souls who say I look younger on the telly should direct their remarks to the BBC's very skilful make-up artists – though I suspect I may be testing even their great skills these days.

No, the reason I am surprised is that, like so many of my friends of a similar age, I do not *feel* sixty-five. I still feel like a young man. In many ways I'm much fitter than I was when I was a hard-drinking thirty-year-old foreign correspondent based in the United States. I can see no reason why I should not be jogging around the park and playing football with my small son and his friends for another few decades. And assuming I have not been sacked by the time you read these lines, I can picture myself still getting up in the middle of the night to present the *Today* programme. I can just about accept the idea that I might one day become bored with doing it, but not that I shall ever be incapable of doing it because I am past it. I simply cannot imagine getting old.

I am, of course, deluding myself. I am confusing old age with 'extreme' old age. As Dr Guy Brown, who works on cell physiology and pathology at Cambridge University, points out, the distinction is crucial. People of my age may help prove that fifty is the new forty and sixty is the new fifty, but there comes a point when that neat little mantra no longer works, however much we might wish that it did. Brown's work shows that an eighty-year-old person today appears to be just as aged as an eighty-year-old several hundred years ago.

And yet the illusion persists that if only we do the right things we can defeat the marauding monster of old age. I blame my own trade: the media. If you listen to the radio, watch the television or read a newspaper it is a racing certainty that in the course of any twenty-four-hour period you will come across some sort of medical story that encourages the illusion. Researchers will have either discovered a miracle cure for some dreadful disease or found that if you eat enough of a certain food it will save you from ever being stricken down by a different but equally dreadful disease.

In the newspapers I read this morning, I learned not only how to survive cancer but also how to avoid heart attacks, the two biggest killers. The cure for cancer lies in eating lots of Chinese food and the way to avoid heart attacks is to drink tea. So that's all right, then. Quite encouraging, really. Except that it is, of course, mostly nonsense. Mostly, but not entirely.

There is (almost) always something in the miracle cure stories and even in the miracle food stories. In the case of Chinese food, for instance, it seems it may well be possible to develop, from whatever it is that gives Peking Duck its orange colour, a drug that might help protect against certain types of cancer. Note all the caveats. There are always an awful lot of 'mays' and 'mights' in these stories. In the case of tea, it's certainly true that it contains natural antioxidants, called polyphenols, which have beneficial effects on all sorts of biochemical processes in the body. The only minor problem is that you have to drink an awful lot of it before the benefits kick in. I've always wondered whether that's why Tony Benn is in such remarkably good shape for a man in his eighties. He gets through about a gallon a day and has done for years. Then again, he does not drink alcohol either, so that may be an even bigger factor. Who knows? The week after you have discovered the miracle food you may very well read a story telling you the opposite. A gallon of tea a day may stop you getting one illness and bring about another. Oh, and stay away from Chinese restaurants if you do not want to die of some ghastly disease brought on by the consumption of monosodium glutamate.

A few centuries ago Newton formulated his Third Law of Motion, which stated that for every action there is an equal and opposite reaction. It is tempting to suggest a similar law for medical 'breakthrough' stories in the modern media: for every positive story there will be an equal and opposite negative. Probably the best thing to do with most of them is to treat them with a large pinch of salt – or preferably a small pinch given that too much salt will kill you. Possibly. Then again, without enough salt we'd die. The trouble is, we do not know which of the stories to dismiss and which to embrace. We can hardly be blamed for that.

Gary Schwitzer is a poacher turned gamekeeper. He was once a journalist and now spends much of his time analysing what journalists do. In June 2008 he published an analysis of five hundred health articles from the mainstream media in the United States. Only 35 per cent of the stories were rated satisfactory on the criterion of whether the journalist had 'discussed the study methodology and the quality of the evidence'. Only 28 per cent covered benefits and only 33 per cent adequately covered harms. The articles routinely failed to give any useful qualitative information in absolute terms. In Britain Ben Goldacre – himself a doctor – writes brilliantly in the *Guardian* every week about the misleading and sometimes downright mischievous coverage of medical stories, not just in the popular press but sometimes in distinguished medical journals whose editors should know better.

Yet even if we dismiss all the miracle breakthrough stories as a load of old rubbish designed to sell a few extra newspapers we are still left with the reality that we are living longer and the question why. Even though the truly great breakthroughs in hygiene, disease control and inoculation happened many decades ago, we are still adding years to our lives with every passing decade. Could it be that our bodies have changed in some fundamental way, that our genes have mutated in a manner that we do not understand? Might there be, in the language of the *New Scientist*, a 'miraculous Methuselah mutation'? Well, if there is, nobody has been able to find it. A more mundane explanation might be lifestyle, which raises another obvious question: how should we live to ensure a long and even happy life?

Most of the answers provided by *New Scientist*

contributors were entirely (and reassuringly) predictable. It helps a lot to have a good relationship with family, friends and even pets. It helps even more to be happily married. At Chicago University researchers found that a married older man with heart disease can expect to live nearly four years longer than a single man of similar age with a healthy heart. Even smoking – the deadliest of deadly health sins – is less likely to kill men who are married than those who are divorced.

On the other hand, we might want to follow the example of the nuns who live at a convent in Mankato, Minnesota. About one in ten of them have made it to a hundred in spite of not being married. Then again, we might not. Being nuns, they eschew all those sins of the flesh in which most of us occasionally indulge. They lead quiet, spiritual lives. They do not drink or smoke, and they eat frugally.

Eating very little is important – and I'm not talking about avoiding obesity, which everyone knows is a big killer. No, the trick is to eat just enough to stay alive. It has been tried with mice, and it works. It has also been tried – after a fashion – with a group of people who ate only three-quarters of their usual amount. By the end of three months they had less insulin in their blood and less damage to their DNA, which is good for longevity.

Something else that has been shown to help us

live longer is having fun and laughing a lot. That may seem to run counter to the experience of the nuns of Mankato, but it doesn't: for all their abstemiousness they are, by all accounts, a jolly lot and enjoy their lives enormously. Tom Perls of the New England Centenarian Study says the one thing that very old people tend to have in common is that they are 'gregarious and fun to be with'.

Being clever helps too. There are many studies which show that if we are fairly intelligent, have a decent education and a good job, we will not only live longer but will be less likely to suffer dementia. But it's important to keep using the brain. A study undertaken at the University of California, Berkeley, has found that playing bridge actually boosts the immune system. Rats which were given maze puzzles to solve and toys to play with lived 50 per cent longer than those which were not.

So much for the fairly predictable lifestyle stuff. What about the science? This is where it gets very unpredictable indeed. This is where we enter the 'death may be optional' territory. And this is where Sarah Jarvis comes in, because on this topic it's better to listen to a doctor than a journalist.

The sense of death is most in apprehension.
Shakespeare

3

Can We Delay the Inevitable?

Ｎone of my patients has ever died of old age – at least not officially. Every time a doctor fills out a death certificate, it lists a main ('primary') cause and then any contributory ('secondary') causes. It is these certificates which give us our national statistics for causes of death.

In the twenty years I have been a GP, filling out death certificates has been a regular part of my job. I have listed heart attacks and cancers aplenty, along with a fair smattering of strokes and lung conditions – but never have I written 'old age'. In fact, it was only when John and I were planning this book that I spoke to the local coroner about the appearance of 'old age' on death certificates, and was told that old age was an accepted cause of death as long as the patient was over seventy-five years old. Apparently, until a few years ago you were allowed to die of old age if you were over seventy, but the rules have now changed. I had heard of 'forty is the new thirty' – but 'seventy-five is the new seventy'? The question is: what actually kills us (assuming it is not entirely obvious, like a concrete block falling on your head)?

It occurred to me only recently that nobody had ever told me that I was allowed to list 'old age'. In fact, it had never crossed my mind to do so. Perhaps my training was in some way deficient? I looked back through our surgery's death certificates and realised that I was not alone – none of my partners' patients had died of 'old age' either. So either my partners are far more skilled than I, or we are all deluding ourselves about the passage of time.

I reckon my practice is pretty representative of GPs as a whole. So why are we failing to exercise the right of our patients to die, on the record at least, for no other reason than that they have worn out? And why, when I think about it, am I so convinced that they are doing just that?

It may be, at least in part, a misguided attempt to give those left behind a reason. No matter how old your loved one is, no matter how frail, dealing with their death is always harrowing. Somehow, it doesn't seem the time for a detailed lecture on the anatomical workings of the miracle that is the human body.

For instance, I often write 'heart attack' or 'stroke' as the cause of death for someone very old and frail who has just collapsed suddenly, clutching their chest, or fallen over with one side of their face drooping. That may be strictly true, but often the reason for their heart attack is that their kidneys have gradually stopped filtering fluid properly, so they retain too much water for their heart to cope with. And perhaps one of the reasons their kidneys packed up was a side-effect of the tablets they needed to keep their heart going. And so on. The medical explanation (for want of a better word) is that the person gradually wore out – but somehow a heart attack is easier to explain.

So the statistics we get from the death certificates are anything but perfect. But what are the alternatives? The only way to know for certain what caused somebody's death is to do a post mortem examination. This might make the death statistics a tad more accurate, but it certainly wouldn't help the person who has died, and can cause untold distress to the family.

Strictly speaking, I don't know what kind of cancer my mother died of (although, admittedly, I do at least know she died of cancer). In fact, I don't even remember what the doctor put on her death certificate. To me that didn't matter, because the only reason for putting a name to the cancer was to put a name to the cancer. It wasn't actually going to extend her span on earth, or improve her quality of life, one jot.

It's not just me and my fellow doctors who like to put a name to what kills us. When I first became a GP, I remember many times trying to explain to the family that grandma or mother had just faded away. 'Yes, we know that,' would be the response, 'but what did she die *from*?'

So why are we so determined to have our lives – and our deaths – neatly pigeonholed and categorised? Perhaps it's all linked in with our determination not to think about death – it allows us to kid ourselves that if we live 'healthy' enough lives, we might live for ever. After all, heart disease is the biggest killer – so we eat our fruit and veg, take cod liver oil and run five miles a day. Cancer is the second biggest – so we don't smoke, and stuff ourselves with antioxidants. And so on. As long as all these conditions have a name, we can kid ourselves that we can escape their clutches – but no matter how we try, we can't escape old age.

John ended Chapter 2 by suggesting that doctors know far more about the science of the human body than the average reader, which is probably true, but we can be every bit as guilty of ignoring the facts. Even after years of training and experience in general practice, we can still succumb to the temptation to look at the patient in terms of the disease, not of the whole person. The temptation is especially strong when you have a patient who constantly turns up with different complaints, none of which ever turn out to have a physical cause. Two minutes into their latest catalogue of symptoms, you can think of nothing but how to reassure them about this problem, too. I had been a doctor for over ten years when Mrs R reminded me of the consequences of this 'can't see the wood for the trees' approach. Mrs R was a heartsink.

'Heartsink' is not a term you will find in any medical dictionary, but every doctor knows exactly what it means. You don't need to catch sight of them: just seeing the receptionist adding their name to your list of patients makes your heart sink. They always have at least one thing wrong with them, and it's always something vague ('I hurt all over') or at the very least illogical ('Every time I wiggle my left toe, I get a stabbing pain in my right ear'). Sometimes it's clear from the start that it's all in the mind, but that doesn't stop the patient coming back once a week to tell you how it's ruining their life. And when one condition does finally settle, it's promptly replaced by another – equally vague, equally debilitating.

Some heartsinks are hypochondriacs, but the two terms are not interchangeable. Hypochondriacs are convinced that every symptom they have means they're about to drop dead of an incurable disease. Unlike heartsinks, however, many hypochondriacs are easy to reassure, at least until they develop their next 'life threatening' illness. What's more, I often like my hypochondriac patients and it is easy to sympathise with their mental agonising. By definition, no doctor likes a heartsink.

Heartsinks manage to make us feel powerless. No matter why doctors go into medicine and a career – whether out of a naïve desire to 'help people and make the world a better place' like some white-coated Miss World contestant, or simply to earn a living – there is something hugely satisfying about success. In medicine, success comes from working out what's wrong and helping the patient get better. But heartsinks, no matter how hard the doctors try, steadfastly refuse to improve.

Another problem is that heartsinks, like hypochondriacs, do get genuinely ill. The internet has brought with it an epidemic of 'cyberchondria' – its sufferers are patients informed (or often misinformed) by 'red flag' symptoms which mean they could be suffering from something nasty or even fatal. Take chest pain. If it's like a tight band, it could mean a heart attack, so that's a red flag. If it's sharp and stabbing, and worse when you cough, it's probably a muscle strain. In the 'good old days', when only doctors had access to medical textbooks, patients rarely knew what the 'red flags' were, so they could not imagine they had them. But these days, the average heartsink is not worthy of the name unless he or she has a full house of 'red flag' symptoms at least once a year.

Mrs R was both a heartsink and a hypochondriac, but not on her own behalf. Her imagined medical ailments all afflicted her husband. He would be marched into the surgery with monotonous regularity to display his swollen legs or his chest – 'He gasps for breath in his sleep, doctor' – or whatever other appendage his wife had declared the latest casualty. She was completely obsessed with his health and he had no say in the matter.

So when I received a message, as duty doctor in the middle of morning surgery, that Mrs R had called, I did not grab my stethoscope and rush to the emergency. Her husband, the message said, was asleep, but had suffered a disturbed night. After dealing with the two unbooked patients from the waiting room, I took a deep breath and returned her call.

Mrs R answered the phone in a whisper, so as not to disturb her sleeping husband. At first, she told me, she had been relieved that he seemed to be sleeping so peacefully – 'He suffers dreadfully with his legs, doctor, and he hardly gets a wink of sleep as a rule.'

When he had failed to rouse himself by mid-morning, she took him a cup of tea and tried to wake him. At this stage, she realised that, while he had never been a snorer, he usually shifted in his sleep every few minutes. 'It's not at all like him, doctor, to lie so still.'

I tried hard not to be irritated. It was the third call that week from Mrs R, and the previous two had been about her husband's inability to get a good night's sleep. Poor sleep was a constant refrain concerning both of them. She had once rung the duty doctor at 4 a.m. because she couldn't sleep, wanting to know if a cup of hot milk would make things better or worse. Now, for a change, he was sleeping well, and this too was apparently a cause for alarm.

I had been half listening to her for several minutes before realisation began to dawn. Mrs R was complaining about her husband's health for the very last time, and she had no idea. My heart sank for a very different reason as I told her I would visit straightaway.

When I arrived I found her husband lying still beneath unwrinkled sheets, silent and very, very cold. We must have talked about his health for hours in the previous month alone, but it had never crossed either of our minds that he would actually die. Yet dead he was – the one medical condition his wife had never claimed for him.

The American statesman Thomas Jefferson had old age all figured out back in 1814 when, at the age of seventy-one, he wrote, 'Our machines have now been running seventy or eighty years, and we must expect that, worn as they are, here a pivot, there a wheel, now a pinion, next a spring, will be giving way; and however we may tinker them up for a while, all will at length surcease motion.'

Medical science these days does rather more than tinker. Some of the advances that doctors see on a day-to-day basis do look pretty miraculous. When I was a medical student, treatment of heart attack within the first few hours consisted of diamorphine, aspirin and keeping a careful eye. Today, this is just the start. We have improved survival rates by almost a quarter with a single treatment – a 'clot-busting' drug injected directly into the veins within minutes of arrival at the hospital. In fact, every hospital now has targets for 'door to needle' time. The drug is so effective, but has such a narrow window of opportunity, that success is measured in minutes shaved off the time it takes to give the treatment.

Drugs like that may keep us alive, but they don't stop us ageing. Once we are past our twenties, our muscles just don't keep their tone the way they used to. The actor Robert Downey Junior summed up the way most of us feel about staying fit as we pass the first flush of youth when he talked about his role in the superhero movie *Iron Man*. 'I'm forty-three, I used to work out for six weeks and look good for six years,' he said. 'Now, I work out for six months, and I look good for six minutes. By the time the other one comes out I'll be forty-five, this is going to start getting really ridiculous!'

It is tempting to pursue Jefferson's machine metaphor. As a machine gets older, it gradually becomes less efficient. Perhaps it uses more energy to achieve the same performance; perhaps it needs more frequent servicing and replacement of spare parts. Eventually, some insult from the outside world pushes it past its limit and it breaks down completely. Each of the systems of our bodies goes through a similar process of ageing. Our immune system, which helps us to fight off infection, ages just like the rest of us. It is made up of a highly complicated mass of cells (called white cells), which travel round the body in a network of hollow tubes called lymph vessels. These cells provide us with the most astonishing defences against the potential invaders which our bodies encounter daily. Made in our lymph glands (six hundred or so 'depots' found at the intersections of lymph vessels), these cells are on constant patrol, primed to recognise an enemy immediately and to call in reinforcements. That, by the way, is why the glands in your neck swell when you have a sore throat – your lymph glands are working overtime producing white cells to fight the infection.

This is no terracotta army – the cells of the immune system are both very much alive and very different from each other. In the main, our immune system is a highly efficient sniper. Sometimes it recognises intruders specifically and shoots them down while it calls for back-up; sometimes it just swallows them whole.

But even the cells of our immune system get old. Our lymph nodes keep producing new cells as old ones die off, but in later life these are less nimble than they were – a Dad's Army. Unlike Captain Manwaring and his soldiers, however, they cannot just be put up for retirement: the new recruits are just as old. Their 'eyes' are not as sharp as they once were, and they jog rather than sprint to our defence. So the odd invader, including the occasional infection, slips past and sets up camp in the midst of the enemy. Germs aren't fussy – they survive just as well in old organs as in young ones – and sometimes they stage a complete coup, with fatal results.

But in the last few decades alone we have defeated diphtheria and smallpox, and we are well on the way to conquering space. Surely the workings of a single human body should not be beyond our control? The trouble is, slowing the rate at which our bodies age involves changing our genetic make-up. To understand why that is such a superhuman task, we need to go back to the biology classroom.

All the functions of our bodies are determined by the make-up of our genes – our genetic building blocks. Sometimes, when we produce eggs or sperm, there are changes in the configuration of these building blocks, called mutations. Charles Darwin's 'Natural Selection' theory of evolution goes something like this. Sometimes random mutations from one generation to the next make us less suited for survival (a mutation which gave you weaker muscles when survival depended on running away from prehistoric predators made it a fairly safe bet that you would not survive for long enough to have your own children and pass that mutation on to them). People who receive this kind of genetic inheritance die out quickly. But sometimes a mutation makes it more likely that you'll survive. Imagine a gene that made your body naturally immune to tuberculosis in Edwardian England. If you had that gene, you'd be more likely to live long enough to have children – an example of the so-called Survival of the Fittest. If that same mutation also helped your children survive, it would spread even further – perhaps two families in the next generation, four in the generation after, then ten, twenty and so on.

The problem with defying death is that we would need to change a lot of our genes. We would need one mutation which kept our joints from creaking; another to keep our brains from wearing out; yet another for our kidneys; and so on. If we relied on evolution, it would take thousands of years for even a single favourable mutation to spread to all of us. It takes centuries, even millennia, for evolution to have a major impact, and medical science means that our expectations have changed within decades.

What is more, a gene that helped us to live longer is not even going to be singled out for special treatment by 'Survival of the Fittest'. For a mutation to spread to all of us, it has to raise our chances of having lots of children, so increasing the number of people who carry that gene. Yet a mutation which stopped our cells from wearing out until we were over a hundred wouldn't have made us more likely to survive long enough to have children. As far as evolution is concerned, there is no advantage in being built for that sort of long-term abuse. As little as a century ago, nobody would ever have survived long enough to take advantage of it anyway. And even if they had, they wouldn't have been better placed to have more children as a result.

So much for evolution – what about our lifestyles? The statistics suggest that, even if we lead absolutely blameless lives, most of us will still run into problems in our eighties or nineties. Sooner or later, things just wind down. In fact, ironically, living 'too' healthily can actually damage our health. Professional rugby players or marathon runners may have healthy hearts, but all that exercise wreaks havoc on their knees.

Of course, that's not to say that we should all just give up on the idea of living healthier lives. The whole point of avoiding risk factors for heart disease is that all too often it doesn't just kill you, it strikes you down prematurely. For instance, almost two out of every five men who die under the age of seventy-five die of heart disease, whereas overall 'only' about one in four men dies of it.

And on the whole, healthy living doesn't just stop you dying of things – it stops you from having to live with them. Take fruit and vegetables. Academics can argue until they're blue in the face (and often do) about whether all the antioxidants in fruit and veg actually do you any good in practice as opposed to laboratory experiments, but studies which involved giving people high doses of antioxidant vitamins didn't stop them dying. But that's not really the point. A high-fibre diet with lots of fruit and veg cuts your risk of dying from heart disease, stroke and cancer of the bowel. But it also stops you suffering the dragging ache and bloating of constipation and the eye-watering pain and embarrassment of piles. The only side-effect? My personal feeling is that wind is a small price to pay.

So lifestyle is hugely important. Even with the best of genes, about 70–80 per cent of the variation between different people's lifespans is determined not by inheritance (nature) but by outside factors during our lifetimes (nurture).

Yet we kid ourselves if we pretend that lifestyle is all that matters. Perhaps we tell ourselves that other people who died of heart disease and cancer didn't have healthy enough lives. Maybe they exercised regularly and didn't smoke, but they did have a weakness for unsalted butter. So all we need to do is to live totally healthily and we can cheat the odds. But to have even an outside chance of living to a great age we'd need to do all the good things and none of the bad, and that would be very dull indeed.

My experience is that people are very good at taking up the advice they like the sound of and avoiding the bits that might be harder work. Of course, what constitutes 'hard work' depends largely on your point of view. For me, a cycle ride at the end of a day's work is the perfect way to brush away the cobwebs – but I can't think of anything more ghastly than a wheat grass smoothie.

What's more, for many things it's not just a question of 'good' or 'bad'. Some 'good' things can be bad for you if you do them to excess. For instance, as a nation the British are many, many times more likely to die from obesity than from malnutrition – and dieting can be an effective solution. Take it too far, though, and you end up with anorexia, which kills you every bit as effectively as diabetes or heart disease, but usually even more quickly.

The same thing applies to medicines. When newspapers report on the huge benefits of some new drug, it is never in their interest to give as much space to the negative as to the positive. By the same token, if they are announcing a 'killer drug', the headlines at least will downplay the number of people it helps. The job of newspaper headlines is to catch our attention, and headlines shouting about 'The New Miracle Cure' sell far more newspapers than statements that 'It will probably save the lives of some readers, but might land a few of you in hospital.' The newspapers often put just the bits we want to see in the headlines, and the boring provisos in the small print beneath.

In the real world, most medicines carry risks as well as benefits. When a doctor writes a prescription, he or she is frequently weighing up whether, for you, the potential benefits outweigh the risks. Take aspirin. It seems that never a month goes by without a new miracle-claiming headline about the humble headache pill. It is remarkable stuff – a daily dose of 75mg (a quarter the dose of a single aspirin painkiller) will cut your risk of a heart attack by a quarter. On the other hand, for every 250 people who take this dose for a year, one will suffer from a bleed in the stomach as a direct result. For every 2000 people who take it, one will die from a bleed in the stomach as a direct result. If you're at high risk of heart disease, these risks are a small price to pay for cutting your chance of a heart attack by a quarter. But if you are young and healthy, and your risk of heart attack is low, taking a daily aspirin may actually do you more harm than good.

The other thing we have to bear in mind is that, no matter how clever we are with the statistics and the science, we still have no idea just how the mind affects our bodies. We know it from experience – John talks about his father 'turning his face to the wall' – and every doctor has seen that happen. The statistics tell us that devoted spouses are more likely to die within the first few months after their lifetime partner's death than at any other time. We can call it a broken heart, we can call it losing the will to live: it still doesn't tell us how it affects our body's vital functions. What is more, it doesn't tell us why. For that, perhaps, we need more philosophy than medical science.

Many of my elderly patients have simply stopped getting a buzz from being alive. It's not just that all their friends have died and they're lonely; it's not even that they are in constant pain, or riddled with arthritis that stops them getting out. They've simply had enough. Dr Johnson may have said that if a man is tired of London he is tired of life, but as far as some of my patients are concerned it can be summed up even more generally: 'If you are tired of living, you are tired of life.'

So much for the science. Living healthily will certainly improve your quality of life, but it can only do so much for the quantity. If we want to die well, we have to accept that we are going to die. And so must doctors. We in the medical profession have to come to terms with the fact that we cannot 'save' everyone. And that means we must stop teaching trainee doctors that death equals failure.

61

Birth, copulation and death. That's all the facts when you come to the brass tacks.
T. S. Eliot, *Sweeney Agonistes*

4

Is Death a Medical Failure?

In all my time as a medical student, nobody ever came out and admitted that they had let a patient die. That, we were told, would be 'giving up'. In fact, I never encountered death in any context except one of failure. As recently as the 1980s, when I began studying medicine, palliative care was in its infancy and the 'science' of medicine was wholly occupied with curing.

There is no module at medical school on dealing with failure – more's the pity. As students, we learn endless details about the path of the ulnar nerve and the physiology of the hypothalamic-pituitary axis. After all, goes the thinking, it may very well come in useful if we become surgeons or endocrinologists. Indeed it may, but only a tiny proportion of medical students ever go on to work in one of these rarefied specialities. All of us, on the other hand, are sooner or later going to have to explain to someone that there is nothing more we can do to cure them. And nobody shows us how to do that.

At least half the thirty-six thousand GPs working in Britain today trained twenty or more years ago.

In those days we spent all but a few weeks of our training in hospitals. We did get some experience of failure – but usually only in the 'morbidity and mortality' meetings designed to examine what are described as 'adverse outcomes' and to learn how to avoid them. These meetings were all about making improvements or changes to prevent mistakes being repeated.

But even at these meetings the concept of failure stretched only as far as blame. If it turned out that a particular death had been unavoidable, the team moved on to the next case on the agenda. No one ever considered pausing to discuss how those looking after the patient felt about the fact that they had not been able to save that person. This may have something to do with arrogance and the stereotypical comedy-show view of the doctor as God. When I was a medical student ritual humiliation was the standard approach. I still remember a particularly bruising teaching session with a surgeon who seemed to revel in showing up my ignorance. As I sat close to tears, one of my friends passed me a piece of paper on which she had scribbled: 'What's the difference between a surgeon and a physician? A physician only *thinks* he's God.' It certainly seemed that way to me then.

In those days, most of the senior doctors who acted as our role models were male. In teaching hospitals competition was fierce, and working over one hundred hours a week as you clawed your way up the career ladder was the rule. No allowances were made for having a life outside the hospital. As a result, all too many brilliant female doctors found it impossible to juggle the conflicting demands of home and work.

I still remember, after forty-eight hours without a break, being called to the cardiac arrest of a forty-five-year-old man. As I went into auto-pilot, trying to bring him back to life, all I could think was 'I don't care what you do – die or recover – as long as you do it quickly. I have to get some sleep.' The next day, I thought seriously about finding another career.

While I was training, more than one consultant made it clear that he didn't know why he bothered to waste his energy on us women. After all, we were going to run off and have babies or (just as bad) become GPs. General practice was what you did if you just couldn't hack it as a 'proper' doctor.

I suppose, in retrospect, it was hardly surprising that in this macho environment death was an admission of failure – and failure was for wimps. I'm quite sure the consultants who taught me had families. Presumably, although we never saw them, they also had feelings. But none of their students was ever given the faintest hint that this was the case, and certainly not that the consultants' own experiences, whether professional or personal, had any impact on their decisions.

Of course we didn't always succeed in curing people, and there were occasions when patients did die on us. Now and again the doctors were pragmatic, and let an unconscious patient who had suffered a stroke slip away quietly. But it was like a guilty secret: we never spoke about it.

Even then, there was a difference in attitude between the surgeons and the physicians. Obviously, some people who are generally unwell are treated by surgeons, but often the surgeon is seeing a patient who is otherwise in the prime of life. Healthy young women go down with appendicitis. Students part company with their motorcycles at 100 miles an hour. The focus was firmly on fixing and the excitement-loving surgeons were 'fixers' to a man.

The future physicians, on the other hand, were more likely to be the cerebral types: the academic nerds, who got their kicks out of pitting their brains against a disease. On the whole, those who practised as physicians were the ones who came face to face with chronic, incurable disease – with patients whose whole bodies had been ravaged by illness. Even if they dealt with one problem, there always seemed to be another to take its place. Perhaps it was only natural that, when they were teaching us, they spent most of their time showing us their medical successes. The subtext was clear. 'If you hang on my every word and work hard enough at being like me, one day you too will be able to work miracles.'

This was not the way I imagined my future life when I announced at the age of eight that I wanted to be a GP. I still remember the day. My father was ill in bed (an almost unknown occurrence) and the doctor came to our house. My mother fussed round the important visitor, keeping me out of his way, but I couldn't resist peeking round the bedroom door to watch him at work. Out of the Aladdin's cave that was his Gladstone bag came all manner of strange instruments and finally, to my enormous excitement, a needle and syringe with which he proceeded to give my father an injection.

The doctor spotted me and called me in, taking me through the tools of his trade – stethoscope, blood pressure monitor, ophthalmoscope – with patience and good humour. Initially in awe of this figure of authority, I had absolute faith that now he was here my father would be all right. After all, that was my only experience – if you were ill, you saw the doctor and he solved the problem. The fact that my father was on his feet within days after the doctor's visit only cemented that belief.

Before he left, the GP handed me the used needle and syringe – unthinkable in the health-and-safety-conscious age we live in today – and my career path was assured. For years, I kept the needle carefully sheathed in an old sherry cork, bringing it out to inject my teddy bear with Ribena. The needle has long since gone, but the bear remains, witness to my amateur attempts at surgery when he developed straw-rot from the injections, and sits on a high shelf in my study to remind me of my roots.

My single-minded determination to be a doctor from such an early age was a source of interest, and sometimes mild amusement, to my parents' friends. I would be wheeled out at parties to declaim my passions: 'I want to make people better.' It would be twenty years before I even conceived of my equally crucial twin role – helping people to die well.

When I was training it was quite normal for the family of a seriously ill patient to be taken to one side by the consultant once the ward round was finished. If the outlook was poor, the relatives would be asked how 'heroic' they wanted the doctors to be in their attempts to save him if, for instance, his heart stopped. The medical students were never, ever invited to join private discussions.

If these conversations were difficult for the doctors, they must have been impossibly painful for the families. It was probably right that they took place in private. These days medical students learn from role play with actors about breaking bad news. But when I qualified there was no such option, and our exclusion from the encounters (real or manufactured) kept us one more step removed from the chance to see death as part of the real world of the doctor.

Medical training has changed a lot over the years, but even today's newly qualified doctors are encouraged to believe that failure is not an option. The only exception is in specialist palliative care, which has blossomed in the last few decades to provide hope for thousands of patients and their families every year. Here, for the first time, medical students learn that it is possible for people to have an active choice in how, if not when, they die. The trouble is that during training the average student spends five years in the 'go-for-it' atmosphere of the hospital, and only a couple of weeks in a hospice.

I recently found myself sitting on a train next to two young doctors who were obviously on their way to London to take their membership exams for the Royal College of Medicine. Throughout the journey, they talked about nothing but the finer points of the possible cause of double vision related to damage to the central nervous system. As I listened, I found myself impressed by their technical knowledge (most of which I had forgotten) but couldn't help wondering if they knew anything at all about human nature. Never once in three hours did they talk about the patients who suffered these conditions as people. They were diseases on legs.

But these were doctors bent on a hospital career, and for those of us in general practice, at least, priorities have changed. We are actively encouraged to talk to our colleagues about how consultations with patients make us feel, and the effect they have on how we treat the next patient. We talk openly about the limits of 'conventional' science, and the profound effect of intangible skills such as looking at problems from the patient's perspective. Newly qualified doctors going through further training to become GPs spend months examining the way they communicate with patients, how well they listen and how much they take the patient's concerns into account. As well as their hospital training, they spend at least a year shadowing a single GP trainer before they are let loose on their own. Here, they encounter patients when they are well – as people with families, dreams and fears. Here, they visit dying patients in their own homes, working in teams with the astonishingly dedicated individuals who make up the hospice community teams that I shall say more about later. In hospital, they have learnt that we are 'conquering' the heart disease and cancer that used to kill people quickly. In general practice, they learn about the flip side – that some people just spend much longer dying.

Much of this change has been driven by attitudes in society. No longer (thank goodness) are patients prepared to do what they are told without reason. We may groan at buzz words like 'empowerment' but most GPs, and many hospital doctors, relish the chance to have a grown-up discussion with their patient about what really matters.

But this shift in attitudes has also been responsible for other changes in the way doctors and patients interact, and not all for the better. Twenty years ago, if the doctor suggested 'letting him go quietly' it was taken for granted that everyone was acting in the best interests of the patient and trying to save him unnecessary distress. Nobody considered whether legal action for breach of human rights or withholding information would be the consequence. But that was then, and this is now. In the last two decades, we have rushed headlong into a blame culture. If someone has died, it must be someone's fault. This means that the spectre of litigation hangs over every healthcare professional. Sometimes it feels as if the law and common sense are mutually exclusive. All too often, when it comes to a choice between the two, human instinct is the casualty.

It is a huge issue for us, and an immensely complex one. We face legal, moral, ethical and emotional problems that our predecessors could never have contemplated. And the biggest ethical dilemma of all is this: just because we *can* keep people alive, does that mean we *should*?

Learning to live with failure is tough. Recently, the doctor I'm training to be a GP gave Mrs M anti-inflammatory tablets for pain. Every doctor knows that this particular kind of painkiller can, very rarely, cause kidney damage. It's much more common in people whose kidneys are not working properly in the first place. This lady's kidneys had been struggling for years, but she couldn't cope with the side-effects of any of the other medication we had tried, and she couldn't cope with the pain.

We started with a tiny amount, hoping to find a middle ground where the dose was big enough to relieve her pain but not high enough to tip her into severe, potentially fatal, kidney failure. We failed. Mrs M's kidneys stopped working, and she ended up in hospital for a week while they recovered. The doctor berated himself for 'giving the patient kidney failure', yet his prescription had also given the same patient the first blissfully pain-free week she had known for a decade. No matter how I tried, I couldn't console the doctor by reminding him that he was doing his best in an almost impossible situation. Finally, I took him to see the patient and we sat down to talk about it. Mrs M was stunned. Surely the doctor understood that she would have done anything to relieve the pain? After all, had she not begged him to put her out of her misery at all costs? My wise patient took this terrified young doctor's hand, looked him in the eye and said, 'You had two choices – give me a treatment, when we both knew the risks, or leave me in agony. Giving me the treatment doesn't make you a bad doctor.

Not giving me anything would have made you a bad human being.'

And there's the rub. Part of every medical student's teaching is '*Primo non nocere*' – first do no harm. But what happens when failing to 'do' is also harmful? Almost every day I watch the doctors I teach grapple with the consequences of their action – or their inaction. All too often, their perception is of being stuck between a rock and a hard place. Certainly when they first encounter the limits of medicine, the hospital way (treat the disease at all costs) may seem a less complicated alternative.

But there are times when pulling out all the stops may not simply be failing to cure the patient, it may be killing them. And sometimes – just sometimes – accepting that a patient is beyond your help might save their life. Medical treatments may have advanced in leaps and bounds over the years, but we are still short of miracle cures that have no side-effects. On the whole, the more powerful the medication, the greater the risks. Think chemotherapy versus paracetamol.

Mrs M is one of the luckier ones. She was seventy-two when diagnosed with heart failure. At first, we set to with gusto to treat her breathlessness and swollen legs. All too quickly things began to go wrong. Her kidneys, it rapidly became apparent, were temperamental performers, and their response to all our attempts to rid her body of excess fluid was a potentially life-threatening work-to-rule.

The pendulum swung back and forth, back and forth. Too much fluid on board ... into hospital with heart failure ... get rid of excess fluid ... back into hospital with kidney failure. And so on. Mrs M's life was turning rapidly into a ghastly round of ambulance trips and hospital stays, with little to come home to. Long divorced, she lived alone and had fallen out with her only son, Derek, who lived in America, many years earlier.

One of Mrs M's many likeable characteristics was her honesty – about her own faults as well as those of others. She was only too aware that her son had inherited from her the pride that prevented either of them from picking up the telephone to re-establish contact. The youngest of three girls, she admitted freely that she had been demanding of her only offspring, unused to the unruly behaviour of 'that peculiar race called men who are put on this earth to create mess for us to clean up'. At the age of sixteen he had dropped out of school to become a drummer. This was most definitely not in the game plan. It was only the first of many disagreements, which had culminated in his marrying a 'most unsuitable girl' ten years earlier. She did not go to the wedding, and they had not seen each other since.

Mrs M was falling into depression. Nothing we did was good enough, and she seemed to hold me personally responsible for her plight. She had always been sharp-tongued, but her inflammatory comments used to be tempered by a mischievous grin. No longer. The district nurses saw her behaviour as a reflection more of fear than of frustration, but her neighbours were less charitable and she rarely had visitors, either at home or in hospital.

I decided she needed to recognise that her time was probably short, and make some decisions about her priorities. Each time we rushed to 'cure' her of her latest complication, we seemed to cause another. She needed to decide if that was what she wanted for the rest of her life.

It was not a conversation I was looking forward to, but in retrospect it was the best thing I could have done. Suddenly Mrs M had a purpose. The moment I mentioned the hospice, her face brightened. Did that mean she could cancel all her hospital follow-up appointments? I was not allowed to leave until I had sat down and explained exactly what each of her tablets did, so that she could get rid of all but the most essential. She rang her son, who immediately offered to visit. A month later, when a place became available at the hospice day centre, she postponed it because he was coming to stay with his family. She met her grandchildren for the first time and took great pleasure in letting them have races through the park pushing her in her wheelchair. Life, she announced, was much more fun now that it didn't matter if she toppled over. Even Derek's wife turned out to be far less than the disaster she had imagined. Donna was, she admitted with a twinkle in her eye, 'Positively charming – for an American.'

But perhaps most surprising – to me at least – was the physical, rather than the mental, change. Once she stopped expecting us to 'cure' her, she became much less impatient and was happy to taper any new treatment to see how it suited her. Within weeks, the pendulum had stopped swinging. Her legs were not as slim as they once were and she couldn't walk up the stairs; but she was stable. And that is the way she has stayed for the last year.

All was going so well until a few weeks ago, when the hospice nurse rang to tell me we appeared to be a victim of our own success. Mrs M was thriving at the hospice day centre and was the life and soul of the patient sessions. But that Monday, she had sunk into an apparent decline after an informal coffee morning at which the staff had outlined plans for their autumn activities. For the rest of the week she had said scarcely a word, refusing to take part in the quizzes or the art classes she had loved so much. When the nurse took her to one side, Mrs M admitted the cause. She was terrified that the hospice would discharge her now that she was failing to get worse. The nurse had tried her best to reassure her that this would never happen and she thought she'd succeeded, but would I mind popping round to check?

I decided to visit unannounced. While she was ill I had seen her at least once a week, but had tailed my visits off when she started doing so well at her day centre. When she opened the door, her scowl told me that she was anything but happy. But as she uttered her greeting, 'Oh, it's you, stranger. I thought you'd forgotten me now that I've stopped dying fast enough', I saw her lip curl in a familiar half-smile. Mrs M was back.

As a GP trainer, one of the most valuable lessons I pass on to the doctors I teach came from a hospice nurse I worked with. She could, she told me, sum up in a single sentence both what being an effective end-of-life carer meant and the fundamental difference between hospital and hospice.

The sentence? 'Don't just do something – sit there!'

After two decades as a doctor, I know that I still don't always get the balance right, and I deal with death on a daily basis. How much more difficult, then, for my patients nearing the end of their lives or, indeed, for their families. When do they accept the inevitable and come to terms with death?

As we will see later in the book, there is a thin line between 'not giving up' and railing helplessly and impotently against fate. The former can prevent a miserable and needless early demise; the latter can make a peaceful end nigh on impossible.

He will live badly who does not know how to die well.

Seneca

5

A Good Death

I may not have Sarah's experience, but I suspect we can all agree on what is a bad death: slow, painful, desperately fearful right up until the end. A 'good' death is more difficult to define. If you had asked me when I was a brash young man for whom death was no more than a vague theoretical concept I'd have summed it up in one word: 'quick'. I might have prefaced it with 'mercifully'.

Don't we all want death to come when we're looking the other way? An enjoyable evening out with friends ... strolling home and sharing a laugh ... then keeling over. And that's that. Dead of a heart attack before you hit the pavement. Or, even better, going to bed one night after a pleasant dinner with the person you love most in all the world and simply not waking up in the morning. Perfect. No pain. No months spent in hospital waiting for the inevitable. No crippling stroke that leaves you reliant on others for everything. Robbed of independence. Robbed of dignity. Above all, perhaps, desperately scared. A sudden death must surely be an infinitely preferable alternative.

That's what I had always thought. That's what I had always wanted for myself in those morbid moments when I contemplated my own mortality. I now think I was wrong. It might be perfect for the person who does not wake up in the morning, but it is a savage blow to the loved one left behind.

Anyone who has not had that experience and doubts the numbing agony it can produce should read Joan Didion's memoir *The Year of Magical Thinking*. It describes in exquisitely painful, unflinching detail the death of the man she had loved for forty years and the effect it had on her. One moment she and her husband were settling down for the evening in their New York apartment, sharing a drink, preparing to eat dinner. The next moment he was lying dead on the floor. He'd had a massive heart attack.

The book describes the year that followed and how Joan Didion dealt with her grief. There were times when she remembered with joy and gratitude the life they had shared together, and there were times when she simply got on with things. But there were the other times too when the grief was almost – though never quite – unbearable: 'Grief comes in waves, paroxysms, sudden apprehensions that weaken the knees and blind the eyes and obliterate the dailiness of life.'

Didion would have grieved for her beloved husband whatever the circumstances, but to lose him without warning, to be so utterly unprepared for the greatest loss imaginable, proved almost too much for her. We all grieve at the death of a loved one, but a good death helps the grieving process immeasurably. The death of Sarah's mother was a good one.

You know the drill: 'Poor old Bill ... fearing the end. I'll never forget where I was when I got the call.' It was one of those 'Where were you when you heard Elvis Presley had died?' moments (scrubbing carrots in the kitchen of a restaurant in Truro where I was working in my school holidays, in case you're interested). My daughter had just turned six, and had finally convinced me that she was old enough to have a loft bed. I was wedged under the half-constructed bed with a screwdriver in one hand when the phone rang. Without thinking I reached for it, forgetting that I was supporting the base of the bed with my other hand. The perilous arrangement collapsed – and so, moments later, did my world.

It was my father. That was the first sign that something was wrong, because it was always my mother who made social contact, with me and everyone else.

'Sarah? I've got some news about your mother, and it's not good. We don't know anything for certain, but she's got an appointment with the cancer specialist for the results tomorrow, and she thought you'd like to know.'

Like to know? The Great British art of the understatement. I couldn't take in the news at first: I'd seen my mother only a week earlier, and she hadn't said a word.

Eighteen hours later I was sitting on one side of my mother, my father on the other, while the consultant gave us the devastating news. My mother had cancer throughout her stomach – they didn't know where it came from, and he didn't want to put her through unnecessary tests to find out. It was too far advanced to make any difference.

How many times had I sat opposite my patients, trying to find the right words for the worst news in the world? How often had I tried to imagine how awful it must be for them to hear? However bad I'd thought they were feeling, I knew now I was wrong. I could never have imagined how unspeakably awful those words were.

Tears were flowing freely down my cheeks, and I felt my mother's arm round my shoulder as she murmured to me that I mustn't worry – it really wasn't so bad. She reassured me that she'd done everything she wanted with her life, apart from seeing my children grown up and married, and she had no regrets. She was ready to go.

After a moment, I realised that at first I hadn't been remotely surprised that my mother was comforting me. After all, I had just had the worst news possible, and looking after other people was what she did. Through a haze of tears, I looked over at my father. He appeared completely impassive, but I knew better. My parents had been married for almost fifty years, and they had one of the strongest relationships I had ever seen. They complemented each other perfectly.

My father was a proud retired army officer, whose main fault was a failure to appreciate that his endless reminiscences were not quite as riveting to his relatives as they were to him. Soldiers were much like children, he used to inform us – as long as they knew exactly where they stood and who was in charge, you couldn't go far wrong.

My mother had been that rare creature, an independent career woman in the aftermath of the Second World War. Tall, fit and tanned, she trained as a sports teacher and went on to represent Northern Ireland at squash. But when she met my father at the age of thirty-six (shockingly, he was a mere twenty-nine) she turned her back on her independent life without a thought.

Throughout her married life, she followed my father from army base to army base, working when she could fit it around his commitments and always, always putting his comfort first.

My father's job, we children were constantly reminded, was very important, and her main aim in life was to make his world run smoothly. As a child, I never realised that there were men who didn't have their afternoon tea brought to them on a trolley within minutes of their return from work. I'm not sure I ever realised men were supposed to know where the kettle was, let alone the washing machine – I know my father didn't. He and my mother had fixed domains: my mother organised the home, the social calendar and the birthday presents; my father the garden, the home repairs and the day-to-day finances. When she was admitted to hospital for an operation at the age of fifty-five, my mother was hugely impressed when he visited the first evening and announced proudly that he had cooked himself scrambled eggs and cold ham. Four days later – when it became clear that every meal had comprised of scrambled eggs and cold ham – she discharged herself early to look after him properly.

Yet my parents actually had the most equal of relationships: a partnership in every sense. All the major family decisions were made by them together as part of the same team. I know my mother never regretted her decision to give up her 'first' career. Her role in their shared life was, she believed, just as important.

She had never been able to get pregnant, and because she was forty-three when she and my father adopted me I always thought of her as old. It was only later, when I saw photographs of her in her youth, that I was reminded of John Betjeman's 'Miss Joan Hunter Dunn, furnished and burnished by Aldershot sun'. My mother was a superb tennis player, and I could easily imagine my father as the infatuated subaltern of the poem. Forty years on, when I caught him studying her, he still sometimes had the look of a man who couldn't quite believe his luck...

As we walked out of the hospital, my mother was already getting us organised. In complete contrast to me, she was calm, unshocked and almost cheerful. She needed a routine, she decided, and she needed things set up so that she could stay at home to die. By the time we reached home half an hour later, she had picked my dazed brain for every possible eventuality and how she could make sure it didn't get in the way of her plans.

For the next few days she seemed essentially unchanged. I returned to work for two days and cleared my diary apart from unbreakable engagements in the audience of my eight-year-old's school assembly and my six-year-old's prize evening. Very little trumps being a daughter – in fact, being a mother is, to my mind, the only exception.

By the following weekend she was already getting weaker. The GP arranged for a hospital bed to be delivered and set up in the dining room for the time when she could no longer manage the stairs. Her biggest anxiety was that she was no longer strong enough to cook my father's supper. I spent much of the weekend preparing meals, labelling them with microwave instructions and essential warnings ('Do not heat this up in the oven – the container is plastic') and storing them in the freezer until my next visit three days later.

During the weekend I was passing the door of their bedroom, where she and my father were resting, when she heard me and called me in. She needed, she informed me, some moral support. She had just been taking my father through a list of the widows in the village, and they thought they'd come up with the obvious choice. But now she realised that this woman was a bit of a disaster in the kitchen. Didn't I agree that, no matter what her husband thought, he really shouldn't marry a woman who couldn't cook?

Over the next week she faded fast, and by the following weekend could only hobble from her bed in the dining room to her chair in the sitting room with two of us helping. But her mind – and her mood – remained as bright as ever. The house was filled with a regular stream of visitors from the neighbours in the village, and it was my father who had to limit the length of their visits as my mother began to tire visibly.

By the third week she was confined to bed – but it was a bed in the home she had built with my father, and even the furniture was full of memories. The dining table around which the family gathered on every major occasion of my childhood was squashed to one side of the room, covered with medicines. The vast oak sideboard they had found twenty years earlier in the yard of a junk shop in Belgium, adopted by the owner's chickens to build their nests, loomed majestic against the wall.

We didn't get it all right. Because she had deteriorated so fast, for instance, her regular medication hadn't been reviewed. She had developed thrush, a fungal infection, in her mouth and gullet, which made swallowing intensely painful. For several days, my father obediently sat with her while she forced down her daily tablets, at a time when even ice cream and water were a major effort. It was only when I was charged with giving her the morning tablets, and realised that each one took several minutes – and huge effort – to swallow, that I took an objective look at what they were for. They included a statin tablet to reduce her cholesterol – wise forward planning to prevent a future heart attack for the healthy eighty-three-year-old she had been a month before, but laughably unnecessary now. By the time I had weeded out everything she no longer needed, there was little left for her to take.

That last Sunday was a glorious English spring day. Sun streamed through the French windows in

the dining room, from where her bed looked out
on to the garden which she had cultivated lovingly
for so many years. The room was full of daffodils
and there was no smell of death. Instead, it smelt
of the aromatherapy oil I used to massage her dry
legs while she sighed with innocent pleasure at the
feeling.

All of us were there. While my brother, my
father and I shared stories around her bed, her five
grandchildren ran screaming round the garden. My
husband and sister-in-law rushed after them, pursued
by the dog. The thrush in her mouth made it hard
for her to speak, but she listened intently despite
the pain she was now in. Early in the afternoon she
asked for a camera, and shakily took photographs
of the grandchildren in the garden – we developed
them after she died.

By mid-afternoon it was clear that she was, for the
first time, in severe pain. The GP, who had visited
in the morning, had arranged for the Macmillan
nurse from the local hospice to visit and fit a pump,
which would release a slow stream of diamorphine.
Before she arrived, my mother said her goodbyes
to the grandchildren. Each one was hugged with a
strength hard to believe from the frail, pale woman
on the bed. She knew, if they did not, that this was
a last goodbye.

The Macmillan nurse arrived, efficient but
compassionate, in the late afternoon. She explained

to my mother that she would need to have a catheter put in once the pump was in place. My father and I stood on either side of the head of the bed, holding her hands. As the nurse started putting the catheter in, she looked up at my mother to check that she wasn't finding it too uncomfortable. My mother replied that no, she was just fine, and that the nurse should continue to 'do whatever you want down there'. Then she turned to me and motioned for me to bring my head closer to hers. She was grinning as she whispered, 'I don't know if I've told you, dear – but it would never do to tell your husband that.'

Late that evening she was sleeping peacefully. We had teased her good-naturedly for years about her snoring: she had a habit of nodding off after supper on the sofa, snoring until her head lolled forward and she jerked awake, always proclaiming, 'I was just resting my eyes.' Somehow it seemed only right that she was snoring gently now. I left my father and brother with her, driving back to London for my son's school assembly the next morning.

I had planned to return as soon as the assembly was over. But the next morning, at 7.45 a.m., the phone rang again. It was my father. 'Is that you, Sarah?' he queried. 'Your mother's just stopped snoring.'

Why was my mother's death so good? Well, obviously, luck played a part. No matter how well prepared you think you are, disasters can happen. The tumour could have broken through the wall of her gut, making her vomit up blood. It could have spread to her brain, making her have a fit. We can never be completely prepared for the unexpected.

But many people die badly from exactly the same condition as my mother. What was it that allowed her death to bring more of a smile than a tear to my eye as I write about it five years later? Mostly it was not what happened – it was how she, and the people who loved her, reacted to it.

My mother came from a generation which saw death as a part of life. She was born in 1919, the youngest of six children, and grew up the only girl, an adored little sister to the five brothers who all died before the age of seventy. Her mother had told her of her own childhood, when one in four children was dead before their first birthday and four out of five never made it past the age of sixty-five. So for my mother, reaching the age of eighty-three was an unimaginable luxury.

Nor did she expect a miracle cure. If anything, she fought less hard against the consultant's stark words than I did. She had lived most of her life as the wife of a soldier who had fought for his country in Korea. She had lived through the Second World War as a young adult, and knew from bitter experience that nobody is immune to death.

Had she really achieved everything she wanted in her life? If she had stopped to think about it, I'm quite sure she could have produced a list of things she had always secretly yearned for, but not had the chance to experience. But that was not my mother's way. It's not that she had led an unusually privileged life, indulging her every whim – money was always a worry, despite a lifestyle that was modest by most people's standards. And it's not that she lived only for the present – more that she knew how to be content with her lot. I suppose the best way to describe her attitude to her end was realistic.

In fact, she actually told me that she thought she'd been extraordinarily lucky in her diagnosis. She didn't want to be one of those people who don't have a chance to say goodbye. For her, those three weeks were just enough to get her affairs (including my father's future marital prospects) in order, but not so long that her illness made her tired of living.

The GP and Macmillan nurses were a huge help. Even though she only had one visit from the nurse from the hospice, we all knew that they were on our side, and ready to step in at any time. Just knowing they were only a phone call away helped her – and us – so much.

I'm quite sure that having her grandchildren around her when she was dying was a great comfort to my mother. In our sanitised society, some people might find it macabre that I was prepared to 'expose' my young children to death. For my part, I think it was just as important for them as it was for her. They were able to tell her how much they loved her, and they still remember that last goodbye. We have had long discussions about the gift of 'loving and losing' rather than 'never having loved at all', and about the comfort they brought her. It may not have been easy for them, but my children have learnt that there is no cure for being dead. And in my mind, if we want to die well, that is a lesson we all have to learn.

If my mother had been much younger, perhaps with a young family, she would have had every right to feel hard done by when she got her diagnosis. I cannot imagine I would have been so pragmatic if I thought I was being robbed of the chance to see my own children grow up. But although my mother still loved her children dearly, she knew she was not the most important person in their lives. That honour went to their children, and this was the natural order of things.

I hope that in some small way her family's attitude helped, too. It's not just that she knew we would be there for her until the very end: many people have that security, but still die badly. It's certainly not that we didn't mind losing her, because we did. But we knew how important it was for her to accept her own death. And if we couldn't prevent it, the best way to help her was for us to accept it, too. Begging her not to die would not have kept her alive – but it could well have made her feel guilty about leaving us.

To a father, when a child dies, the future dies; to a child, when a parent dies, the past dies.

Red Auerbach

6

The Trouble with Families

A bad death is much more likely if we don't get the chance to prepare or if we refuse to accept that life isn't always fair. But there's more to it than that, and it's not just down to us. Most of the good deaths I have seen as a doctor have involved the whole family working towards exactly the same end – singing, if you like, from the same hymn sheet. I've always admired families who are absolutely determined to let their loved one decide how he or she wants to die. As far as they are concerned, if the star of the show knows what they want, the family's only job is to help them get on with it.

Why do I admire them so much? After all, surely what they do is only natural. Don't we all want to do the best for those we love? Sadly, doctors in practices like mine know differently. Doing what you think is best and doing what your relative wants are not necessarily the same thing at all. That's why it is so crucial not just to think about your own end, but to engage your family in the bigger picture. If you don't, there is a real risk that protective instinct, rather than pragmatic acceptance, will take over. I, more than most, should know how disastrous that can be. I have seen exactly what happens if your relatives try to ride roughshod over your wishes in a misguided attempt to 'do the right thing'. I have watched Agnes die.

Agnes H ('You're more than welcome to call me Agnes, dear, but nobody calls me Aggie twice') was eighty-one years old with a wit – and a sharpness of mind – that would put many twenty-year-olds to shame. She had been rushed to hospital with severe stomach pains caused by a complete blockage of her bowels. Although she was fully conscious when she arrived, there was little doubt that without surgery she would be dead within days.

Despite this, Agnes was anything but keen to be operated on. She had, she told me, lost her husband of nine years after routine surgery. He had had an aortic aneurysm (a swelling of the largest artery in his body), and although it had never caused him any symptoms he was told that it could burst at any time. The only permanent solution was major surgery, but this too could lead to complications.

Agnes and Douglas had met through their local church two decades earlier, a year after Agnes was widowed. They had agreed that he would carry on working until Agnes retired, to increase their pension and let them indulge their shared love of travel by taking a world cruise. They discussed the risks of the operation at length: after all, it was their retirement, as well as his health, at stake. Finally, they agreed it was a risk worth taking – she couldn't bear the thought of losing him suddenly at any time.

But lose him she did – and slowly. Douglas suffered a stroke during his operation, which paralysed him down one side and left him incapable of speaking clearly or looking after himself. He had to be fed and changed like a baby, and Agnes regretted most of all the loss of his dignity. Eight months later he died when his kidneys failed. He had never reached home in the interim, although she visited him daily in the hospital and then in the nursing home. After his death, she did not go into a terminal decline but confided from her hospital bed that her grandchildren – and, indeed, everything else in life – offered only a fraction of the joy they once did.

As her pain increased, Agnes finally agreed to an operation – with one stipulation. If the blockage was caused by incurable cancer, she should be 'closed up and sewn up and jolly well left to get on with it. I may not have any choice about whether I go under the knife, doctor, but I'm far too old to be the subject of any pointless heroics. I know what you lot are like when you get your hands on a challenge, and I won't have any of you picking through my insides trying to work out what belongs and what doesn't.'

Sure enough, Agnes's obstruction proved to be caused by cancer, with cancerous seeds spread like debris after a hurricane. She was moved back to the intensive care unit and, although she came round from the operation, her kidneys, too, began to fail.

Initially she was not in severe pain. That popular medical catch-all description of 'poorly but comfortable' covered her condition perfectly. But she was adamant that she did not want any further procedures which would be designed to prolong her life. She wasn't scared to die: in fact, she was far more scared to carry on living without her beloved husband.

Agnes was a highly intelligent, if not highly educated, woman. Her arguments came from instinct and determination, but her logic was flawless. What she really wanted, she admitted, was for us to 'give me what I'd really like to end this nonsense'. She knew we couldn't do that – she knew we weren't allowed – but she also knew we couldn't cure her. We couldn't even prolong her life without the risk of leaving her in the same state as her husband had been. And that, she announced firmly, was not an option.

Agnes's daughters had been at her side constantly since she came into hospital, and had listened quietly to her persuasive demands to be left alone. They didn't try to change her mind and later, in the family room, they admitted that they were only too aware that the 'spark had gone out of her' since her husband's death. All too often they had heard her confide her horror of his prolonged final months of suffering.

The same could not be said of Agnes's son. He swept in two days later, loud and obviously angling for a fight. Agnes was dozing when he arrived and he did not even wait for her to wake up before he demanded a meeting with the doctor to talk about 'this "I don't want any treatment" rubbish'.

I was not the senior doctor on the team so I was only a silent observer, but the anger in his body language was hard to miss. Here was a man used to getting what he wanted – and what he wanted was to haul somebody over the coals. How dare we, he asked, take such a decision upon ourselves on the say-so of a sick and distressed woman. Had we not considered that, ill and weak as she was, she had no idea what she was saying? Call ourselves doctors? We just wanted to make room in the intensive care unit for someone younger. All right, he eventually conceded, his mother might not have years of life left, what with the cancer and all, but he was damned if he'd let the doctors discard her like some substandard reject at quality control. What was more, he wasn't prepared to take our word that she knew what she was saying. He wanted a second opinion.

His sisters sat silent. Their rationale, they admitted later, was that if they spoke up he would simply make his arguments directly to their mother, and she had always found it harder than anyone to cope with him when he was in one of these moods. They apologised on his behalf to the doctor. For the four decades since he had left home, his parents would hear nothing of him for months on end. Then suddenly, without warning, he would swoop in with extravagant presents or harsh criticism of how his sisters were looking after them. 'Well, it was guilt then and it's guilt now,' was his sisters' succinct summary of the situation.

Sadly, every doctor has had experience of the family member motivated by guilt: they are always the ones who shout loudest and complain most bitterly. They are also the ones most likely to sue. We all knew perfectly well that Agnes knew precisely what she was saying. She was also more than capable of convincing any judge. What was more, she was perfectly entitled to refuse treatment even if we, or her son, had been convinced she should have it. But Agnes's son would not be suing until after she died. And that meant we would be missing our star witness.

So we agreed to talk to Agnes about a formal assessment from a psychiatrist which her son had demanded without telling his mother. The moment we broached the subject, she snorted with laughter. 'He's got to you, hasn't he? He thinks I've lost my marbles. Well, I'd rather be carted off to the Funny Farm than let those surgeons at me again. In fact, you'd better stop all my medicine first – don't want him claiming my answers didn't count because I was all drugged up.' So Agnes had her assessment and passed with flying colours. She knew exactly what her decision meant: she would not be leaving the intensive care unit alive.

The long process of assessing her mental state – and particularly the lack of pain relief – took their toll, and Agnes was fading fast. It was proving harder to bring her pain under control again than it had previously been, despite our best efforts. So we were not entirely surprised when, the next evening, her son demanded another meeting. What did surprise us was what he wanted. This time he had decided that we were inhuman to let his mother suffer so much and something must be done to help put her out of her misery. Again I stood in the background as he raged – his face red, the veins on his neck standing out, his belly quivering with righteous indignation. Couldn't we just give her an injection to let her slip away quietly? He wouldn't tell anyone if we did – he couldn't bear to see her in distress.

I could hardly believe what I was hearing. Yesterday, apparently, we had failed when we didn't engage in futile heroics to save his mother against her will. Today we were guilty of refusing to kill her.

Agnes and I had spent hours chatting in the wee small hours. She had, it seemed, only one major anxiety about dying. She had been married twice and knew that both her dead husbands would be waiting for her when she 'arrived'. She and her first husband had been keen dancers ever since their courtship, and her second husband was also 'silver-toed enough to keep all the girls on the dance floor green with envy at me'. There was one question nagging away at her. When she arrived in Paradise, which one should she dance with first? She had loved them both and was consumed with anxiety that one of them was bound to feel let down.

Between us, we reached a conclusion. Douglas had known when they met that she had been married before and loved her in spite of this. In fact, he had often told her that her obvious devotion to her first husband had been one of the first things that attracted him to her. Here was a woman who loved with a fierce passion and loyalty, so wouldn't it be the best feeling in the world if he could prove himself worthy of that love, too? Of course Douglas would understand that she must give the first dance to her first husband. She would not have been the woman he married if she didn't.

She returned to this subject on the fourth night after her admission. By this time, her kidneys had all but stopped working and the toxins in her body were building up fast. Her breathing was becoming laboured and even a few moments of conversation were enough to tire her. Over the course of the next four hours she drifted in and out of sleep. Every time she awoke, she complained of pain and asked that the dose of her diamorphine infusion be increased.

I reminded her only once that the levels of painkilling medication were now reaching the stage where they might cause her problems with breathing. She smiled and replied, 'Do you really think I didn't know what you are and are not allowed to do?'

The last time she awoke, she seemed much more comfortable. She called me over and we talked about how much less guilty she felt about that crucial first dance. Before she drifted off to sleep for the last time, a smile played about her lips and she tapped her fingers on the sheet.

'Do you know,' she mused, 'I'm beginning to hear the music.'

Now it is time that we were going, I to die and you to live; but which of us has the happier prospect is unknown to anyone but God.

Socrates (having been condemned to death)

7

Facing Up to Reality

The prospect of dying holds such horrors that we may be tempted to 'protect' our nearest and dearest from the news. Twenty years ago, I regularly saw the senior doctors in hospital talking to the family first. We had discovered that the patient had, say, a tumour that was too advanced to operate on. We couldn't cure him, but treatment such as radiotherapy or chemotherapy could give him some extra time. The trouble was, these treatments came at a cost. There was the sickness and the loss of appetite; the tiredness and the baldness. What did the family think? Was it better to tell him about the options, and risk making him give up all hope when he knew his condition was hopeless? Or should they just leave him in blissful ignorance and make his last days as comfortable as possible?

Those days, on the whole, are gone and I for one am very glad. I am convinced that all patients have a right to know they are dying. Sometimes they make it clear when we talk that they don't want to think about it, and of course I respect that. One of my patients, who has lung cancer, refuses to think about the fact that she will die from it. She won't say the word 'cancer', and we have agreed a sort of code. I'm allowed to talk about her 'thingy' – as if it's an irritating rash, or a mischievous child – but never her 'cancer'. I'm not sure if she even admits it to herself, but that is her choice.

Mr S never had that choice, and I will always regret that. When I first met him I was a junior doctor and he was fifty-four, a police sergeant with a wife and four children. He had a blockage of his intestines, which the surgeons found was caused by cancer. At his operation, it quickly became clear that there was no point in trying to remove it – it was far too advanced for that. But they relieved the obstruction, and when he came round from the anaesthetic he was no longer in pain.

In the meantime, his family had been told the bad news. They were adamant that the truth should be kept from him: 'Forget the cancer, the shock would kill him.' While my consultant nodded agreement at their comments I stood in the background, far too low-ranking to interrupt and ask why they were so sure he wouldn't want to know.

As a junior doctor you spend most of your time on the wards, getting to know each patient – far more time than the consultant, who breezes in every day with his retinue to spend five minutes at the bedside. Yet nobody ever asks for your opinion – or, at least, they didn't twenty years ago. Your job is to take the bloods, write up the medicine charts, answer questions in the way your consultant has decided. And that, when I was looking after Mr S, was what I did.

But Mr S was persistent. As I stood by his bed, checking on his progress, he would tell me about his family but also ask me about his condition. I tried to be suitably vague about the cause of his blockage, but doing so felt so uncomfortable that I even plucked up courage to ask my consultant whether we should talk to the family again – I was convinced that Mr S was suspicious. He said no, and I never spoke to the family myself. Three days later I was writing up a chart at the next bed when I overheard Mr S talking to two of his children behind the closed curtains.

'Why won't the doctors tell me what's going on?'

'What do you mean, "what's going on"? There's nothing to worry about.'

'I'm not going to die, son, am I?'

''Course not, Dad – we'll have you home in no time. Now don't you trouble yourself. After all, you've got to save your strength so you're well enough to walk Claire down the aisle.'

'Yes, you're right. But you will tell me if you hear anything, won't you? There's so much I want to tell you all before I go.'

Half an hour later, I passed them in the corridor. They were discussing whether they should tell their father the truth. But Claire, the soon-to-be-married daughter, was tied up all that day, and their brother James the next. It would be three days before they could all sit down with their mother. They would talk through the options then and decide. It was only right that they should make the decision together. After all, it was too important to decide without all of them having their say.

In the event, it was Mr S who never had his say. He developed a blood clot on the lung, and died the next day. He never had the chance to share the 'so much I want to tell you'. Perhaps there was nothing the family didn't already know – but the point is, he didn't have the choice.

Some of us, of course, are going to die suddenly: no warning; no time to dwell on what we wish we'd done. But if we never think about dying we may be tempted to keep putting off the fun things in life, possibly until it's too late. When I was training as a GP, the senior partner in a neighbouring practice was the epitome of the dedicated old-fashioned doctor. For forty years his family came second in his priorities, as he gave himself body and soul to looking after the patients who knew him affectionately as Dr Jim.

His wife told me she had lost count of the number of family occasions he had missed because of an urgent visit to a sick patient, which always seemed to take longer than he'd expected. Of course she was proud of his dedication, but she didn't think it was too selfish to want a bit of him for herself. She yearned for the day he would finally retire. They were planning to move closer to their children, miles away from his practice and the temptation just to 'pop in' on old patients even after he had hung up his stethoscope.

The day finally came, and Dr Jim seemed relaxed and content. He allowed himself to get caught up in the excitement of the move, and the prospect of spending more time with his grandchildren. Within weeks he was killed in a car crash, so Dr Jim never did get his retirement. Deaths like his are untimely and tragic – but they happen. As so many lifestyle management websites on the internet remind us, nobody's last words have ever been: 'I wish I'd spent more time at the office.'

There is a world of difference between knowing you are going to die and accepting it. To have a good death like my mother's you must have not only a supportive family and good medical care, but the ability to make the most of the chance to say goodbye.

The American country singer Tim McGraw wrote a soulful song about being diagnosed with incurable cancer, in which he talks wistfully about the joy of having the chance to 'live like you were dying'. If we spend all our lives convinced that our time will not come any day soon, we are less likely to be able to grab that opportunity. Nor are we likely to be able to accept our fate and come to terms with it, even when it is too late to fight. If we cannot accept the inevitable, then neither can our family – and the legacy of that anger is the last thing we want to leave behind.

Mr and Mrs H had always been an unlikely couple, but it was a match which had worked for thirty years. When I first met them I was struck first by their obvious devotion to each other, and next, in fairly rapid succession, by their intelligence, their humanity and their sense of humour.

At first sight, they couldn't have looked more different. She was the picture of middle England. Seventeen years younger than her husband (and looking three decades his junior), she was always immaculately turned out in crisply pressed frocks. Whenever I did a home visit, there was home-made cake with tea in a china cup. She worked with several charities and, with a 'jolly hockey sticks' good humour, cajoled and charmed people she knew into supporting them. He was a lifelong socialist who had spent most of his working life as a maths teacher at an inner city comprehensive. His hair stuck out at wild angles, giving him the look of a mad professor. And in spite of his wife's best efforts, his freshly ironed shirts were always stained with food or cigarette ash. Years of smoking had taken their toll on his chest and he drank far more than was healthy. But his mind was razor-sharp, and he was always ready with a clever answer when I brought up the subject of his lifestyle. I never did make any inroads into his whisky consumption or his smoking.

I suppose I, like everyone else, made assumptions. One day his life would catch up with him – lung cancer, liver failure, maybe a heart attack – and she would be left a widow. Maybe she would occupy her time with her charity work and her grandchildren; maybe she would make a new start and find love again. After all, she would still be young enough and fit enough. Mrs H had never said as much, but it was obvious that she too assumed she would outlive her husband by many years. She was the one who ate her five portions of fruit and veg a day, while he stopped at the chip shop on the way home. She went swimming twice a week; he went to the pub. So when she came in with stomach pains that turned out to be cancer of the pancreas, we both felt it was terribly unfair. The problem was that this sense of injustice took up all Mrs H's emotional energy – and from that moment, there was nothing else in her life.

When the first specialist told her the cancer was too advanced to operate on, she demanded a second opinion and then a third. When the cancer specialist tried – oh, so gently – to make her understand that any treatment could only relieve her symptoms, not cure her, she took to the internet. Day after day was spent searching for ever more exotic and unlikely miracle cures – crystal therapy, coffee enemas, macrobiotic diets and faith healers.

Her obsession with finding a cure left no time for preparing for death – or even for making the most of the life she had left. She wouldn't think of taking a trip with her family; she wouldn't talk about where, or how, she wanted to end her days. Her husband and children admitted to me that they found it almost impossible to find anything to say to her: they were always on tenterhooks, in case she took offence at some innocent remark. They couldn't talk about global warming because she would not be around to witness the consequences; they couldn't talk about the state of the economy, because it reminded her that her husband would need the help of the social services after her death. The children had always had a close relationship with their mother – but now their visits were punctuated by long, awkward silences and polite conversation. Even her friends could no longer offer her comfort.

Mrs H became too weak to keep the house in its usual immaculate state, but she refused to let her children help or even to employ a cleaner. That would be to admit that she wasn't well. And if the house wasn't clean, she couldn't have visitors. Letting her standards drop would also be admitting defeat. So her friends from the local church, the Women's Institute and the bridge club found themselves turned away at the door. Gradually they stopped coming and the house, which for so many years had rung with the chatter of her children's friends or the laughter of social gatherings, became silent.

Ironically, Mrs H did die at home – but more because she refused to leave than because we had planned it properly. I had tried to talk about the options, including visiting the local hospice to see if she liked it. Mrs H looked at me with distaste and said, 'There's nothing wrong with my home. It has served me well for twenty years of married life, which is more than can be said for the hospital or the hospice. I'm not supposed to be in hospital as a patient. The thought of spending my life there as a visitor when my husband's time came was bad enough, but I really won't have any more of it.'

So I worked with the hospice, social services and the district nurses to set up twenty-four-hour-a-day care. I tried to reassure Mrs H that everything would be done to make sure she didn't suffer but, though she listened, I don't think she really heard me. When it came to discussing her wishes for saying goodbye to her family and friends, and her funeral arrangements, my courage failed me. Despite years of experience and training in communication skills, sometimes the right words just don't exist.

Eventually Mrs H took to her bed, now set up in the dining room because her bedroom was too small for her to be nursed in. This, too, of course, upset her. She hated the fact that her lovely dining room had to be vandalised (her word) to accommodate the bed, her medicines and the oxygen equipment. She hated the fact that nobody could clean and tidy to her high standards.

Mrs H fought with all her strength against the cancer – but eventually she lost. And sadly, it was a battle right to the end. She couldn't stand being dirty, but she hated the indignity of being washed by the nurses. She wasn't in pain – we had seen to that – but she resented the fact that the painkilling medicine made her sleepy. Everything should have been right. But somehow nothing was. And because she was so angry and aggrieved about the unfairness of her illness, her family were too.

When Mrs H finally faded away, her husband and children were by her side in the home she had lived in for twenty years. While it should have been a textbook 'good death', in fact it was anything but. There was no comfort for her family, when all they remembered was her suffering.

And their troubles did not end there. Even though he had survived his wife, Mr H was still a sick man and now he was a bitter one, too. He refused to leave his home and move in with his children, but rattled round in a house that was far too big for him to cope with. He hated the endless stream of carers who were never going to live up to his wife's standards. 'To think that I should be reduced to relying on *people*,' he announced once when I was visiting, the seemingly innocent word dripping with venom 'when I should be enjoying a happy retirement with my wife. She would never have let it come to this.'

Most of his carers refused to come back after a few days. His barrage of insults scared them, and when one persisted he barricaded the door to keep her out. He sat inside the house with the curtains closed and his beloved jazz music turned up to full volume. When the carer continued to bang on the door to attract his attention, he called the police to report an intruder. Mr H's son, summoned by the carer from her mobile phone, arrived at almost the same instant as a panda car with sirens blaring.

And so, with his wife gone, Mr H became a recluse. He refused to let his children take him to the pub, and he refused to let his friends come to him. Like her, he just faded away – and as with her, it was horrible to watch. Five months after his wife's death, he failed to wake up. This time when I visited, to certify his death, the conversation with his children was very different.

Gradually they opened up about their own grief at the family milestones their mother would not be around to share – the younger child's wedding, the first grandchild. Their mother had been the glue which held them all together, but because their father was suffering so acutely from her untimely death their own feelings had to be put on hold. It was only when he too was gone that they were allowed to grieve not just for him but also for her.

It's hard not to be affected by our own experiences. If we've seen somebody we love die badly, we may subconsciously feel that there is nothing we can do to prevent ourselves from suffering the same fate. Perhaps we have seen human misery on a grand scale, and protected ourselves by inventing a fairytale scenario for our own end. Or maybe we've worked with dying patients and the attitudes of a bygone era are fixed in our psyche for ever.

But death, like life, has come a long way in a few short decades. Britain leads the world in palliative care, and every day brings new solutions to the problems dying people have been grappling with for centuries. If we are realistic about what we are facing, and what we want most to avoid, there is a good chance of getting things right. But the doctors and nurses who deal with dying are not mind-readers. How can they know what we dread most if we don't know ourselves? And how can we know if we are not honest with ourselves?

Philip Jones Griffiths had seen more than his fair share of death during his professional career, so you might have expected him to take a realistic view of his own when, at the age of seventy-three, it became clear that his life was nearing its end. Yet his attitude came perilously close to denying him the good death he so richly deserved. Philip had become a good friend as well as a patient. I knew that he had been a brilliant photographer and a campaigner for the human rights of the innocent victims of war. These entries posted on the internet give some idea of the respect in which he was held:

> Of the photojournalists I truly admire, Philip's photos were truly remarkable. He left an indelible mark on the history of photography, the history of the world and most importantly, the history of man.
>
> Philip's iconic work on the Vietnam War ... is arguably the most articulate and compelling anti-war statement made by any photojournalist ever. Indeed it led Noam Chomsky to comment that: 'If anybody in Washington had read that book, we wouldn't have had these wars in Iraq or Afghanistan.'

But the one I am most proud of – and the one which at one stage I never thought would be written – was this:

> Philip enriched all our lives with his courage, his empathy, his passion, his wit and his wisdom;

and for many he gave to photojournalism its moral soul. He died as he wanted so passionately that we should live – in peace.

When Philip was first diagnosed with cancer, his response was predictably brusque. Pol Pot hadn't stopped him telling the world about the worst excesses of despotism, and neither would a mere tumour. The fact that the tumour had already spread, making permanent cure unlikely, was a minor inconvenience. He seemed to accept that one day 'My luck will run out – but when it does, I'll get myself on a plane to Thailand, sit on a beach and take some opium when the pain gets too bad.'

And for seven remarkable years his luck held. His trips would be fitted around his courses of chemotherapy, and there was no time for convalescence in his packed diary. I looked forward enormously to his visits to the surgery, when we would 'get the boring medical stuff out of the way' before he regaled me with tales of the incredible courage and humanity of the people he had met.

The first real setback came when he was struck down with pneumonia on a trip to the furthest reaches of Cambodia and his life hung in the balance for weeks. It was months before he was fit to fly back to England and his breathing never recovered, though his mind remained as sharp as ever. He was back at his computer before he had even unpacked.

Come to think of it, he never really unpacked. In all the years I knew him, I never visited without picking my way between the suitcases and the rolls of film; there was always another book to finish, another injustice to tell the world about.

About three months before he died, it became clear that his tumour had stopped responding to treatment. Even then, he refused to curl up and give in. Indeed, if anything the news strengthened his resolve. He informed me, in a matter-of-fact tone, that he would stay at home to die – he would go into the hospice if strictly necessary, but under no circumstances would he die in hospital. He proposed to write his last email with whatever energy he had left, to allow his family to help him into bed, and to go to sleep for ever.

For a few weeks, it seemed that he was well on track for the perfect end. He had started taking steroids to relieve his breathlessness, and was delighted that they gave him insomnia. He described the steroids happily as his 'mother's little helper', giving him a few extra hours in the day (or in his case, the night) to get on with his work before his time ran out.

One Tuesday, I went straight from visiting him to a clinical meeting at my practice. Every month the doctors and nurses discuss all the patients on our End of Life register, to make sure that all of us know their wishes and how their condition might change and can step in at any time. It's also a great chance to talk about problems with accessing services or getting equipment: someone around the table is bound to have done battle with that particular layer of bureaucracy before.

I like to think I'm not superstitious, but I do wonder if I tempted fate that day. The visit had been everything I could have wished and I was positively upbeat about Philip's prospects. He had, I reported happily, set his affairs in order, accepted that this time he wasn't going to recover and decided exactly how and where he wanted to die. His family, spread all over the world, had dropped everything and moved in to look after him. They were everything I would have expected from his relations – caring, intelligent, unflappable. I reckoned that his chances of getting the end he wanted were excellent.

Two days after the clinical meeting, it all went dramatically wrong. After his pneumonia, Philip had suffered clots on his lung and, to prevent this from happening again, had been taking Warfarin tablets to thin his blood. But a side-effect of the medication is an increased tendency to bleed, and Philip's nose started bleeding with a vengeance. We had no choice but to send him into hospital for an operation to stem the flow.

Three days later he was home again, much weaker and very, very scared. It quickly dawned on all of us that Philip had not really come to terms with his own death at all – he had only come to terms with the stressless, almost fairytale ending he had conjured up in his imagination. Until now, he had managed to convince himself that if he was determined enough he would die as he had imagined – with no pain, no blurring of his mental faculties. He knew he would get more breathless and more tired; but as far as he was concerned, sooner or later he would press 'save' on the last image from his book and go to sleep for good.

The relatively minor medical emergency had jolted him out of his fantasy and he had to come to terms with death all over again – but this time in far more realistic terms. Watching him grieve for his own life made it all the harder to tackle his wishes about his last days. It was clear that everything he had said about how and where he wanted to die was based on this fantasy. And with time running out so fast, any one of these issues could become crucial at any time. We needed to know what Philip wanted, and we needed to know before it was too late.

So every day we tackled a different aspect. It was heartbreaking to watch the internal struggle. With every new topic I felt I was throwing the cruel reality of his imminent death in his face again. Did he want to stop his Warfarin? His initial response was anger: stopping his medicine, he felt, was tantamount to throwing him on the rubbish heap. But if he carried on, he could have another bleed at any time.

Did he really want more active treatment? Even though he knew that more chemotherapy or radiotherapy would not cure him, he still clung to the hope that it might buy him a few precious months or weeks of life. But it was productive life he wanted, and chemotherapy almost always has side-effects which would be even harder for him to cope with than most because he was so weak. He might get an extra couple of months – but it was more likely to be two months of living death rather than any meaningful life.

Did he want to be resuscitated? The ambulance service would be obliged to pull out all the stops if his family panicked, called them out and they found him pulseless. But cardiac resuscitation is anything but the miraculous reviver the medical soaps would have us believe. It fails more often than it succeeds at the best of times. In Philip's case, there was not a chance that it would succeed – and the drama on our television screens rarely reflects the distress that this least peaceful of ends can cause to the helpless family.

Did he definitely want to die at home, or was the hospice still an option if necessary? Here, Philip was completely immovable. Before he went into hospital, he had said he was prepared to move to a hospice if it was the only way to ensure he had a peaceful end. Now he was solidly against it. Anything but dying at home would be a defeat.

Unfortunately, his home could hardly be less well suited to terminal nursing care. His globe-trotting lifestyle, and his ceaseless concentration on his work, had meant that his one-bedroom flat had always come way down his list of priorities. Every corner was crammed with film containers, computerised editing equipment and archive files. Getting him in a wheeled office chair (he refused a wheelchair) from the sitting room to the bathroom involved clearing a path through the piles of paperwork on the floor, and lifting him and his chair up and down rickety steps. Almost the whole floor space of his small bedroom was taken up with a low futon – not the easiest of beds to sleep on, let alone to be hoisted up from.

Tentatively, I broached the subject of adapting his flat, or at least of organising the equipment that the nurses would need to turn him, bath him and change the dressings on his legs, swollen and weeping from the long hours sitting still and upright at his computer. He had told the family he wasn't prepared to think about it. If his home were turned into a hospital, it would compromise his precious work. Painfully, indirectly, we danced around the harsh facts – a hospital-type bed might get in the way of his work, but without some sort of compromise he couldn't stay at home at all. Yet again, reality had to intrude on the illusion.

Until now, every discussion since he had come out of hospital had been a sparring of minds, which felt more like a battle for supremacy than true partnership, but at least we had reached agreement on every other small change. Yet here he drew the line. A hospital bed was for dying in, not sleeping in. We explained that he did not need to start using it straightaway – it would take a few days to arrive once it was ordered – but it was still, in his mind, one step too far.

We were stuck in an impasse until his daughter came up with an inspired compromise. We could install the bed, which could raise him and lower him electronically to a sitting or lying position, in his study. He could keep his own bed in his bedroom and, if necessary, one of his carers could sleep in the hospital bed until he felt able to use it – or until he had no choice. The turning point came when I pointed out that without it, getting out of bed might take up so much energy that he wouldn't be able to work. You never stop learning in general practice.

And so it went on – two steps forward, one step back. Two days later he was exhausted, having been up all night in pain. We spent yet another hour in a circular discussion about the risks and benefits of strong painkillers.

Phillip had a horror of morphine. He had been a pharmacist before he became a photographer, and informed me on more than one occasion that during that first career he had been responsible for mixing the now old-fashioned morphine mixture known as Brompton's Cocktail. Every time he did so, he confided, he knew that the patient was now past hope. The 'lure of sweet oblivion' offered from morphine swallowed up any who succumbed to its charms, and they started to die from that moment on.

My arguments about medical progress fell on deaf ears. I knew the pain relief would help him if he would just let it. I even talked to his daughter about leaving some painkilling 'lollipops' (literally suckable sweets, laced with fast-acting painkillers, on lollipop sticks) in the house for her to give him. But even though our deceit would have been for the best of reasons, we couldn't bring ourselves to do it.

Finally, not surprisingly, the compromise centred on his work. If he was in too much pain to sleep, he wouldn't be able to function. A small dose of night-time painkiller might mean that he would not have to greet the dawn in a state of pain-addled exhaustion. He agreed, and the next evening I visited to find Philip a changed man. His pain had been entirely banished by the medication and suddenly he was ten years younger – invigorated, enthusiastic, playful. Mildly shocking anecdotes were recounted with vigour, and we giggled not in embarrassment but in delight.

His aspirations and determination, too, had changed overnight. He was, he announced, in my hands: he would follow whatever advice I gave. It was only as I left that it struck me what had brought about this apparently miraculous change. It wasn't the painkillers. It was the fact that he had made a conscious decision to accept his departure. I sat in my car in the quiet streets of west London and wept before I telephoned John. We had been researching the book for three years and I knew he would understand that I needed to talk. No matter how we try to keep up a professional air, don't ever assume doctors are not affected by their patients' suffering.

The improvement lasted for two days. On the third, his daughter phoned me while I was away in Wales to tell me his pain had returned with a vengeance. He was begging her to give him the cyanide capsule left over from his travels in the killing fields of Cambodia, and which was still secreted in one of his rucksacks. I started ringing round my colleagues, desperate to do something – anything – to relieve his suffering.

And it worked. All the advance planning, all the coordination with the palliative care team and the district nurses, proved to be worth the effort a hundred times over. Within three hours, the morphine pump we had hidden at his flat for exactly this eventuality was in place and he was sleeping peacefully. By the time I arrived that evening, straight from the train, he was a man at peace. I offered to visit during the night if he passed away, but his family was adamant that there would be no need. If he died in the night they would have time to say goodbye, and would call me at 7 a.m. so that I could visit on my way to work.

Everything we achieved, we managed because we were a team. The Macmillan and district nurses rose, as they always do, to the challenge. To them, it seemed, there were never problems, only solutions waiting to happen. Every member of Philip's family could give lessons on communication skills. While I would sit on the edge of his bed, leading the discussion about the latest painful subject, they always knew just when to chip in with precisely the right soothing, supportive words. Every one of them must have gone through the full gamut of a lifetime's emotions several times over in those few weeks – yet they never faltered. Philip had a right to be very, very proud.

The next morning, the telephone rang at 7.01 a.m. Half an hour later I was sitting with his relatives on the floor of his study, a proof copy of his last book in my hand, and again tears streamed down my face. I did not try to hold them in for the sake of the family – we knew each other well enough.

Death is not extinguishing the light; it is putting out the lamp because the dawn has come.

Rabindranath Tagore

8

Hope and Consolation

If death is a part of life, it follows that a 'good' death is part of a good life. I wrote earlier that it is difficult to define a good death, but there is one factor on which, I suspect, most of us can agree. Given a straight choice between dying at home and dying in a hospital bed, home wins almost every time – Sarah's mother was lucky in that respect – and politicians have finally woken up to this. I spoke to the Health Secretary, Alan Johnson, about it on the *Today* programme in the summer of 2008 when he announced a consultation on what the government calls an 'end of life' strategy.

Mr Johnson said he wanted to confront what he rightly called one of society's last taboos: how we face up to our own deaths and the deaths of those closest to us. At the heart of the strategy was the idea of helping to make it possible for people to die at home if they wished to do so rather than in a hospital. Incidentally, Mr Johnson also told me he had been warned by his staff that other news programmes that morning had decided not to run the story because it would be 'depressing' for their listeners and viewers. That's not just stupid; it's wrong. Far be it from me to criticise my colleagues, but any editor who regards his listeners or viewers as so empty-headed that they cannot cope with the subject of dying should either pack it in and run an amusement arcade or apply for a job on one of those vacuous lifestyle magazines.

Before talking to Alan Johnson I had interviewed an impressive young woman called Maria Gleeson, who proved to anyone with half a brain that it is possible to talk about dying without 'depressing' any but the most emotionally barren listener. Maria's husband Paul had died at the age of fifty-one from cancer. What she told me was not only deeply moving but life-affirming.

When the consultant gave them his diagnosis he had asked where Paul would go to die, making an automatic assumption that he would choose a hospice and not even mentioning the possibility that he might die at home. That surprised both Paul and Maria, but they were too shocked at the time by the actual diagnosis to question the consultant further.

'We went home and we had no contact with anyone for weeks,' said Maria. Eventually she made what she described as 'discreet contact' with their local Sue Ryder home. By then Paul had talked about dying at home. What the hospice doctor told her convinced her it would indeed be the right thing to do. I suggested to Maria that she had made a brave decision, given the challenges she would face caring for a dying man. 'Possibly,' she said, 'but the doctor gave me the courage.'

The Gleesons had three daughters aged ten, fourteen and sixteen, all of whom played the piano. Maria asked the doctor what she should do with the girls when the time came. Instead of trotting out a glib answer she merely said, 'You will know what to do with them.' And so Maria did.

'The piano was hugely important,' said Maria. 'The girls gave a little concert every last day of their daddy's life. He listened to the music, guided their practice, gave them instructions. And all three children were there when he passed away.'

Did she have any misgivings about her decision? Absolutely none.

'It was the right thing to do. When the children look back, I hope they will remember that they had their last hug literally with their daddy, with his last gasp. They will have good memories that they helped me care for him.'

And for her?

'I was there and we had all that time together. He never had to worry about whether I would leave him at the hospice and what was happening to the girls left at home. I was there whenever we wanted to be together … for five minutes or all night. It was hugely important for me. It felt the right thing to do. I could not have considered being anywhere else.'

And for Paul?

'That's what he wanted: to be at home in his own surroundings, his own smells, his own food, his own children.'

Maria Gleeson's eyes were shining as she spoke. She was still in mourning for a man she had loved for many years, but she knew he had died well and she will always have that to remember.

And the Sue Ryder doctors? They are in the business of helping people to die well in their hospices. You might have expected them to put some pressure on Maria to tell Paul he should be admitted. Not so. Five days before he died, Maria had phoned the hospice to confess that she was 'struggling' and asked for help. The doctor who spoke to her confessed that she should really be encouraging her to think about having Paul admitted to the hospice. But she did not do that, because she clearly felt it would be better for everyone if he died at home.

'She gave me the extra "oomph" I needed,' said Maria. 'She told me, "We can have your husband here, but we can't have your children and we can't have your piano." '

And later, after Paul had died, that same doctor told Maria that she and Paul had unquestionably taken the right decision. She added this perceptive comment: 'We are afraid of death in this country and we should not be. We present newborn babies to the world but we do not talk about the other end of life. We should.'

That doctor was a brilliant example of the modern hospice movement – a movement that has probably done more to help people in the final stages of their lives than any other in history. It was the inspiration of an extraordinary woman, Dame Cicely Saunders.

Cicely had a miserable childhood. Her mother was a cold, remote woman in an unhappy marriage. When she was one, Cicely was given into the care of her Aunt Daisy, who showed her the love denied her by her mother. It did not last long. Her mother was jealous and Cicely was forced to return to her. She was a shy girl, withdrawn and timid, but turned into a tough young woman who was determined to care for others in a way that she herself had not been cared for.

She was a student at Oxford when the Second World War broke out, and she left university to train as a nurse at St Thomas's Hospital in London. The first man she fell in love with was a patient at the hospital: a Polish Jew, one of the few who managed to escape from the infamous Warsaw ghetto. He died soon after they met, and his suffering left an indelible mark on her.

Soon afterwards she worked in a home for dying people, and then went back to St Thomas's to retrain as a doctor. She never had any doubts over which branch of medicine she would choose to specialise in. For seven years she researched the control of pain. After she had qualified, she wrote an article arguing for a new approach to the end of life in which she said, 'It appears that many patients feel deserted by their doctors at the end. Ideally the doctor should remain the centre of a team who work together to relieve where they cannot heal, to keep the patient's own struggle within his compass and to bring hope and consolation to the end.'

She introduced a system of pain control that reversed the old approach, under which patients would almost have to beg for another dose of painkiller when they needed it. She saw no need for them ever to reach that stage. They were given regular relief, and if it resulted in them becoming addicted to morphine her attitude was: so what? They're going to die, so what does it matter if they become addicted? She argued that there was no such thing as intractable pain, only intractable doctors, and if physical pain was alleviated then mental pain was relieved too. As the *British Medical Journal* put it, she distinguished between mild, medium and severe pain, each of which was to be treated differently. She also used medicines to relieve other problems of the dying, including bedsores, nausea, depression, constipation and breathlessness.

By now Cicely had fallen in love with another patient. As before, he was a Polish refugee and once again – in a series of tragic coincidences – he died soon after they met. By then she had decided to set up her own hospice, focusing on cancer patients. She met plenty of resistance from those who believed that euthanasia was the best way to deal with people destined to die a painful death. She thought that was rubbish and said so. In 1967 St Christopher's, the world's first modern hospice, was opened.

Many years later she set out the philosophy at the heart of everything she was trying to achieve: 'You matter because you are you, and you matter to the last moment of your life.' Dying, she said, was a phenomenon 'as natural as being born', and death itself was a process that should be life-affirming and free of pain. She once asked a man who knew he was dying what he needed above all in those who were caring for him. He told her, 'I need someone to look as if they are trying to understand me.' That made a huge impression on her: 'I never forgot that he did not ask for success but only that someone should care enough to try.' She saw dying, she said, as an opportunity to say 'thank you' and 'sorry' to family and friends.

Since then, millions of people around the world have had reason to say thank you to Dame Cicely. Until she opened St Christopher's, hospices were mostly grim institutions run by religious orders where people went to die – usually in pain, and often alone and afraid. Today there are about three thousand modern hospices in the United States alone, caring for a million people. In the United Kingdom there are more than three hundred.

Here is how the *British Medical Journal* described the effect she had on the care of the dying:

> She introduced effective pain management and insisted that dying people needed dignity, compassion, and respect, as well as rigorous scientific methodology in the testing of treatments. She abolished the prevailing ethic that patients should be cured, that those who could not be cured were a sign of failure, and that it was acceptable and even desirable to lie to them about their prognosis.
>
> She put paid to the notion that dying people should wait until their painkillers had worn off before they received another dose, and scotched the notion that the risk of opiate addiction was an issue in their pain management.

In her own words: 'We will do all we can not only to help you die peacefully, but to help you live until you die.'

When my former wife, Edna, was diagnosed with pancreatic cancer in her early fifties I feared for the effect on my daughter Catherine of what would inevitably follow. The bond between mother and daughter is powerful, and they were about as close as it is possible for two human beings to be.

After an exploratory operation the surgeon told us Edna could expect to live no more than three months. She survived nearly twice as long. In fact, 'survive' is the wrong word; it was more than surviving. She lived those months to the full, and in many ways they were good months. As much as anything, that was because of the love and care she had from Catherine, who gave up her career and home in London to move to Wales to be with her mother for as long as it took. It may not be possible to prove it in a laboratory, but I have not the slightest doubt that love is the most powerful drug for someone facing the final challenge.

Those months were not easy for my daughter – a popular, lively young woman in the prime of her life. There were some bad days and even worse nights, when she would spend the small hours comforting her mother, stroking her back, holding her in her arms. But when death came, Catherine knew her mother was prepared for it and so was she.

I said that these were, in many ways, good months for Edna. That is not the contradiction it may appear. She knew her cancer could not be beaten, and she refused chemotherapy or any other treatment that might have given her a few extra weeks or months of life.

'Why would I want to go through all that and be thoroughly sick and miserable for a year when I can be reasonably fit and active for a few months?' she asked the doctors. They agreed. She might have added – and sometimes did: '... and when I can use the time to get my life in order'.

Before the cancer struck she had often said that she would like to go on a sea cruise one day, but when I suggested that she and Catherine should go off on one she wouldn't hear of it. She had recently bought an old dairy in the village where she had spent her childhood and she was determined to finish the job of turning it into a home. Which, of course, she did. She was simply not prepared to die until it was complete and until all her other affairs were 'in order'. So they were busy months and, yes, they were good months.

The Macmillan nurse, who visited regularly, was wonderful. She seemed to have some sixth sense that told her when to call – apparently knowing, wherever she was and whatever she was doing, when Edna needed her most. There might have been some kind of invisible bond between them. Superstitious nonsense? Probably. But Catherine lost count of the number of times the doorbell would ring when her mother was at a very low point and the nurse would be on the doorstep, always knowing what to do to help. Macmillan nurses may not be saints, but many do a pretty good impersonation of them.

The local cancer hospice – Holm Tower in the seaside town of Penarth – was wonderful too. That was where Edna went to die. Before I visited Holm Tower I could imagine nothing more soul-destroying for a doctor or nurse than working in a hospice. Most patients go there to die and you know that, barring miracles that simply do not happen, nothing you can do will change that. The staff never have the joy of seeing a baby born or a sick person get well again. There is none of the glamour of cutting-edge medicine, none of the drama of a brilliant surgeon transplanting a new life-giving organ, no prospect of a lucrative Harley Street practice in years to come. I remember asking the doctor who was caring for Edna – a fiercely bright and articulate young woman – why she had chosen to practise in a hospice. She seemed genuinely puzzled by the question.

'It's incredibly satisfying,' she said. 'The job of a doctor isn't just curing people, it's reducing suffering. That's what we do here. We help people die at peace and in dignity. I can't think of anything more rewarding.' She paused and then added, 'It means so much. It's a wonderful job.'

I know how corny those words look when they're written down, but they did not seem corny to me at the time and they do not seem corny now. A few weeks later I had the privilege of watching them put into practice.

I was in the BBC Westminster offices on a Saturday morning preparing for the *On the Record* programme that I had presented every Sunday for almost ten years. Catherine called to say that the end was near, and I drove down to Penarth.

When I arrived Edna had only a few hours left. I sat in her large room overlooking the grey waters of the Bristol Channel as the sun went down. I had seen a great deal of violent death in my years as a foreign correspondent, but that was the first time I had watched a life ending peacefully. She was breathing deeply and easily. The occasional sigh escaping from her lips was the only thing to suggest that this was more than just a deep sleep.

The room was almost dark when a nurse slipped quietly in through the half-open door. I said nothing and I don't think she saw me in the corner, almost hidden as I was by a half-drawn curtain around Edna's bed. She stood for several minutes looking down at the dying woman. Then she leaned over and stroked her hair, as gently as a mother might caress a sleeping baby. And then she left again. There was nothing else to be done, nothing else she could have done. Before the sun rose again Edna was dead.

Technically, I am told, she was killed not by the cancer but by the drugs. The dose was steadily increased to keep one step ahead of the pain, until eventually her heart gave out. She died – as the young doctor had promised – in peace and with dignity. The doctor might have added something else. She died surrounded by love.

It is hard to have patience with people who say 'There is no death' or 'Death doesn't matter.' There is death. And whatever is matters. And whatever happens has consequences, and it and they are irrevocable and irreversible. You might as well say that birth doesn't matter.

C. S. Lewis

9

The Gold Standards Framework

Regular listeners to the *Today* programme may be surprised when I say this, but I have a good deal of respect for most politicians – not least because, in many respects, it's a rotten job and someone's got to do it. But, like the rest of the human race, I enjoy poking fun at them occasionally and I enjoy it even more when someone else does it well. Perhaps the most famous – if unintentional – put-down of any politician in the last century was delivered not by a brilliant satirist or savage cartoonist, but by a small boy standing with his mother in Downing Street. In those more trusting days there were no barriers manned by policemen with machine guns. If you wanted to take a stroll up Downing Street and pose for pictures on the doorstep of the most famous address in the land, there was no one to stop you. The boy watched the various grand figures going to and fro in their top hats and frock coats (it was many decades ago) and said nothing until Her Majesty's Chancellor of the Exchequer turned up and strode purposefully into Number Eleven.

'Mummy,' he said. 'What's that man for?'

History, sadly, does not record her response. I suppose it's even possible that the whole thing was a figment of some bored hack's imagination. But if it didn't happen, it should have. The small boy's question is one that has been asked in various guises by countless voters over the years. What are politicians for? Yes, of course we know that we need them, just as much as we need teachers or doctors or bus drivers. Democracy would not work without people who, whatever their motives, want to be elected so that they can run the country – or at least oppose those who do the running. But what does that mean? What do they actually *do* for most of that time? How come we don't miss them when Parliament goes into recess for breaks which are so long they make a teacher's summer holiday look like a Bank Holiday weekend?

The cynical view is that when they are not on arduous fact-finding trips to the Caribbean they spend their time plotting and scheming against each other so that they – and not their very dear friends and colleagues – will end up sitting on the back seat of a ministerial car. That is a terrible slander. They merely spend much of their time doing that. When they are not plotting or 'fact-finding' they are working on delivering initiatives. There are unlikely to be any reliable statistics in this area, but if you printed out every political initiative announced over any given parliamentary term you would need a library the size of an international football stadium to house them all.

Most, as we know, end up being dumped long before they get anywhere near the statute book. Many have the lifespan of a mayfly. They flutter their wings briefly on the *Today* programme, for instance, and are never seen or heard of again. A classic example was the initiative that would have allowed police officers to haul young miscreants off to the nearest cashpoint machine and force them to draw out twenty quid to pay a fine on the spot for whatever piece of mischief they happened to have committed. It barely survived a day.

The other intriguing thing about political initiatives is the large number of them that are dismissed out of hand by the people whose jobs and lives they are meant to make easier. This applies especially in education and health. Ask a typical teacher what she thinks of the various initiatives announced (or delivered) over the past couple of years and you will need the heat shield of a satellite re-entering the earth's atmosphere to withstand the blast of fury. It can almost always be summed up in one sentence: 'Why don't they just leave us alone to get on with the job!' It's the same in the NHS.

The cynics have a point – even if one accepts that the poor old politicians and, more specifically, the civil servants and armies of advisers who work for them must be seen to be doing something. How else do they justify their salaries? But we can also sympathise with the teacher who is told by the man in Whitehall to do one thing one year and the precise opposite the following year. Today's revealed wisdom is, as often as not, an idea that was tried out several years ago and found wanting. Or – and this is just as likely – proved successful at the time but was dumped in favour of the latest fad. I have written a couple of books about the idiocy of the 'initiatives' forced on schools in the late sixties which meant that two generations of children were taught no grammar. It has now been reintroduced – after a fashion.

What is truly remarkable and curiously satisfying is how many of the great initiatives over the years have come not from the politicians but from the professionals – the people who actually do the job. It was Florence Nightingale who transformed the nursing profession. It was Marie Stopes who transformed birth control. It was, as we have noted, Cecily Saunders who transformed the care of the dying. The difference is that they were not 'delivering initiatives'; they were mounting crusades.

It would be foolish to suggest that politicians and their initiative never make our lives better with their initiatives, but the medical profession (like teachers) are almost always deeply suspicious of them. The aim of what is known as the Gold Standards Framework was to increase the chance of people getting the sort of death they wanted. Sarah, like most doctors, was sceptical – and, as she now freely admits, she was wrong.

When I first stepped over the threshold as a 'proper doctor' on 1 August 1990, I thought only one thing mattered, and that was making people better. We would be a team: me and my patients. How naïve of me. I should have recognised there would be other 'members' of that team: the Whitehall bureaucrats and their political masters with their own agenda.

In the years since, I have bemoaned the endless targets which land on my desk with monotonous regularity. All too often they have no practical value, satisfying only political expediency. They have improved care in some practices – certainly they help to bring the standard of the lowest up to what most of us regard as 'minimal competence' – but for the majority of doctors their main effect has been to come between us and our patients. The fact is that my practice, like many others, has been working to higher clinical standards than the official targets for years.

The target culture has not changed the quality of care I provide, but it has changed the way I have to record things. If I don't enter the correct code on the computer, the official records don't recognise the work I'm doing and that is a serious problem for someone like me who has been described accurately (if politically incorrectly) as 'technologically blonde'. Every hour I spend checking that I have recorded what I'm doing in the 'official' computer language is an hour that I could have spent talking to patients. But the government's appetite for targets seems unstoppable. You can almost imagine the discussion in the hallowed corridors of Whitehall:

'See your GP the same day? Brilliant idea – that'll be a vote-winner, and God knows the polls are looking grim at the moment. Quick, announce some targets immediately!'

'Err – excuse me, sir – if we force GPs to keep lots of appointments free to see patients the same day, doesn't that mean there aren't going to be as many appointments for patients to book in advance at their own convenience? Doesn't it mean patients will need to see the doctor who's free, instead of choosing to wait to see the doctor they trust?'

'Stupid boy – you have a lot to learn! First, they aren't patients, they're voters. Secondly, time is money – voters don't care who they see, just how quickly they get a service!'

'But what about elderly patients – sorry, sir, voters? What about voters who are dying? Don't they want to see someone they trust? Perhaps we could do a pilot study, to see if it works in real life?'

'Pilots? Pilots, boy? D'you think we're in the RAF? Pilots take time, and that marginal by-election is in six weeks. We don't need a pilot, we need an announcement!'

So on the whole I am not, to say the least, a fan of targets – which is why my passion for the targets of the Gold Standards Framework (or the GSF to its friends) is a surprise to me as much as anyone. But passionate I am – because, unlike so many other targets, the GSF is all about talking with patients.

That's the good news. The bad news is that even the GSF cannot avoid its fair share of tick-box lists. So here goes. The GSF aims:

- to offer people in the last year of life more choice in how, and where, they die
- to help patients to live out their last days in their own homes, if that is what they want
- to cut the need for emergency admission to hospital, by making sure that everything the patient needs to keep them comfortable can be provided at home, and if necessary at short notice
- to support GPs and community nurses, who do not deal with terminally ill patients on a daily basis
- to support family and carers, as well as patients.

So far, so wishy washy? Not at all. Those of us who work in general practice may see far more people dying than the average man on the Clapham omnibus, but they're a tiny minority of the people we look after. Compared to, say, a Macmillan nurse or a hospice doctor, we can go through a professional lifetime and still be novices. And when the care of the dying patient is so fundamentally different from the rest of our work, it can be hard to keep on top of all the changes. In fact, that's why the GSF was set up in the first place – by doctors in general practice for patients in general practice. It came into being only in 2001 and started small, with a few pilot programmes. Today it has spread across the UK, and is gradually being expanded to include people in nursing and care homes, and people with conditions other than cancer.

The longer I spend as a GP, the more convinced I am that including these groups has been a huge step forward in helping us to die well. Other diseases are just as deadly and can be every bit as distressing as cancer. People with heart failure, for instance, have a lower life expectancy and quality of life than many people with cancer, and the older we get as a nation the more common these conditions become. Yet people with diseases other than cancer (including heart failure) are four times less likely to end their days under the specialist care of a hospice.

The term 'Gold Standard' was a deliberate, if not an obvious, choice. When the idea was being developed, patients and carers who were polled expressed a fear that within palliative care there is a risk of throwing in the towel: 'Sorry, but there's nothing more we can do for you.' The term 'Gold Standard' deliberately flies in the face of such fatalism. Even though this kind of teamwork may not always succeed in giving patients the death they want, it will never be for want of trying.

But the aim of the GSF is not just to hit targets and coordinate care. It's also about helping doctors to keep communicating. It may seem like a contradiction in terms. After all, isn't communicating what doctors, especially GPs, are supposed to do every day? Why should we need help?

I'm not ashamed to admit that I often make assumptions about people based on my own subconscious views or even prejudices. When I've had ten patients in a single surgery complaining of a cough and nine of them have been requesting antibiotics ... well, there's a good chance that I'll assume the tenth coughing patient is, too. In fact, he may be there because his father has just been diagnosed with lung cancer and he used to smoke himself ten years ago. He may have convinced himself that his cough is actually the first sign, because he remembers his dad coughing endlessly in the weeks before he was diagnosed. But if the patient doesn't tell me what he's actually worried about, I may never make the connection.

And so it is with dying. We all want to help our patients, and much of what we can offer comes in the form of trust and compassion. It's tempting to stick to the 'safe' subjects, to avoid an awkward encounter that gets in the way of our relationship. It's also easy for us 'scientists' to forget, when we're completely convinced of the effect of a certain path of treatment, that logic is all too often overcome by fear.

That's why, when I'm following the GSF, I have a checklist of practical questions I have to answer. Have I talked to the patient about where they want to be cared for? Do I know where they really want to die, and what might make them change their mind? Have I found out what really matters to them, and have I made sure that everyone looking after them understands this? For instance, one person might find it a huge relief to have someone come in to wash them, while another might find it a horrifying intrusion. One person would rather not know exactly why we're recommending a particular treatment, because too much detail makes them queasy; another might feel like a piece of meat if we just get on with our job without explaining everything as we go along.

Mary Murray had a really good death. I'm proud to say I played a part – but I know that the Gold Standards Framework must take most of the credit.

Mary was the Irish Catholic of folk tales. The oldest of seven children born in ten years, she had been a little mother to the youngest. Her mother was struck down with multiple sclerosis when she was eleven, and from then on she was effectively the woman of the house. She had cared for her mother and seen all her brothers and sisters married, remaining at home and unmarried until she was thirty-one, when her mother died.

Mary moved to England to train as a nurse, a career she pursued until she retired at the age of sixty-four. She lived in an immaculate studio flat in a slightly seedy area of Shepherd's Bush in west London, under a shared ownership scheme for key workers run by the local Housing Association. Two years before she retired, she was diagnosed with breast cancer. After treatment she returned to work, but a year after her retirement the cancer returned. It had spread to her liver and bones.

Mary received the very best treatments – initially with traditional chemotherapy, and later with the new breast cancer 'super drug' Herceptin. For the first three months her symptoms seemed to be improving, but by the fourth month the tumours had stopped shrinking and there was a suggestion that they were even growing. We discussed her treatment, and the likely changes that would be made. I asked her how she felt about the Herceptin. She had been a nurse all her life, she responded, and had too much experience to believe in miracle cures.

Had we stopped the conversation there, my next course of action might have been entirely different. I believed that her training had overcome her faith, even her hope. But the Gold Standards Framework stresses constantly the need to explore what the patient's hopes and concerns, as well as their wishes, really are. So I turned the subject to more general contemplation of the future of medical treatments and cancer 'cures'.

It was at this point that Mary added wistfully, 'Of course, just because I know something is impossible doesn't mean I can accept it. I mean, I know that the drugs I've had so far have been the best ones anyone with my condition could ever have – and I know they still haven't worked for me so far. I also know that if a drug like that hasn't worked by now it isn't going to, and nothing will. But that doesn't mean I want them to stop treatment. I can't stand the thought of that, because it'll make me feel as if they've given up on me. I have a horrible feeling that if they give up on me now, I'll give up on me too.'

Mary's honesty was brave, but it left me with a hopeless dilemma. Fifteen minutes earlier, I had felt genuinely confident that I knew what advice to give. I had been convinced that unless the treatment, with its unpleasant side-effects, was going to work she would feel she didn't want to put herself through any more. Chemotherapy is a serious treatment for serious physical problems. The thought of giving it for peace of mind had not entered my head.

Within weeks, it was clear that Mary was fading fast. She grew weaker by the day and finally chose to give up her chemotherapy. On most of my visits she seemed troubled and listless but refused to admit, despite my gentle probing, that she was feeling the mental stain. She also continued to avoid the subject of who would care for her at the end.

On a few occasions I had visited when one sister or another was over from Ireland, and she was visibly brighter. It was clear that she came from a close-knit family and missed her family's company dreadfully. The trouble was that her small flat was scarcely big enough for her and her possessions, let alone any of her siblings staying full-time. I decided that the time had come to talk to her about her wishes for the end of her life.

Discussing a patient's death is never easy for a doctor, however essential it may be for the patient. Over the years we had talked many times of her love of Ireland and of her desire to retire there to spend more time with her family. Instead, within a year of retirement she was dying in the city she had lived in for thirty years – not in the country she still thought of as home. A decision had to be taken, and soon. For the next few weeks she would be strong enough to travel to Ireland to live out her last days, but after that it would be too late.

The last time I had tried to broach the subject of how long she had to live, she changed the subject abruptly. On the following visit she could scarcely bring herself to speak to me. It would not be an easy conversation, and had it not been for the Gold Standards Framework I would probably have given in to the temptation to put off our chat. One of the advantages of having a structured set of aims is that you have to explain yourself when you fail to meet them. During our most recent clinical meeting at my practice, where we discuss all our terminally ill patients, one of my partners had challenged me about why Mary had not made a decision on her preferred place of death. I was forced to admit that I had been too much of a coward to press the subject.

As I approached the door, I was cursing the Gold Standards Framework: wasn't my job difficult enough already? Little did I realise how it would change Mary's life. Much of a GP's work is routine, almost mundane. We make small differences – often, we hope – to a lot of people. Sometimes we make a fundamental difference to a single patient's life, but it's impossible to know when that will be. Thanks to the Gold Standards Framework, this was just such a day.

This time I refused to let Mary change the subject. I explained that while I was absolutely not giving up on her, we needed to make plans while she was still capable. As I coaxed, tears began to run silently down her cheeks. Finally, between sobs, she told me that she didn't want to think about where she would die because she knew she couldn't go home as she wanted.

'What makes you say that?' I asked.

And then it all came out. Mary had neither the time nor the energy to sell her flat to raise money, and she had virtually no savings. A nurse's pay is modest, and living in London doesn't come cheap. In England her medicine came from the NHS, but in Ireland she would have to pay. Her sisters would look after her, but she couldn't ask them to pay for her treatment. I almost laughed with relief when I realised this was all that stood in the way of her return to Ireland.

Mary and I had been on different wavelengths. She had avoided talking about her wishes because she was convinced that the death she wanted was impossible. I had mistaken her sadness for antipathy, and had so nearly avoided bringing up the subject again. Now months of miscommunication had come to an end. Solutions to all her concerns, arranged with a few simple phone calls and a prescription pad, had always existed.

Her sisters arrived within two days to help her put her affairs in order, and she departed for Ireland with them a week later. Three months' supply of medicine filled a whole suitcase. In the end she would use all but two weeks' worth.

She moved into a bedroom in her sister's home, with views of the mountains from one window and the sea from the other. Her other four sisters and two brothers were frequent visitors, and towards the end took turns to sleep in her room in case she stirred. Two days before she died, she saw the joint celebration of her sister's fortieth wedding anniversary and her niece's wedding. Family and friends congregated in a marquee in the garden, and her bed was rolled out on to the terrace to hear the speeches. I heard from her sisters that she had then slipped away quietly at 'home'. Mary had the death she wanted.

Sometimes, as with Mary, the Gold Standards Framework provides a small push (or two) in the right direction that is enough to transform a death. Often, the help it offers is more concrete. Mr Y was one such example.

He had arrived in Britain some seventeen years earlier, an asylum-seeker from Vietnam. Although he had never learnt much English, he had managed to find work as a builder's labourer within a few months of his arrival and had been in full-time employment ever since. The Vietnamese community in west London was small, and his long hours at work meant he never managed to fit in language lessons. Consequently he was socially isolated, living alone in a rented one-bedroom flat.

Despite this, he was always cheerful, polite and pleasant. The doctors and nurses at the surgery met him twice a year to monitor his high blood pressure, but it was not until the practice gained access to a Vietnamese interpreter, some eight years after he had registered, that we learned about his background. He and his wife and child had left a life of grinding poverty and political repression, risking their lives to reach the promised land. There they had been promised regular work, prosperity, safety from indiscriminate violence and torture, and a secure future for their children. The work (and the safety) had transpired, but only for him. His wife and son had been struck down with typhoid on the boat crossing, and their bodies had been thrown overboard by the crew.

When Mr Y was fifty-two, he collapsed at work. He was admitted to hospital and diagnosed with a tumour of his spinal cord. Although the immediate problem was treated with surgery, his long-term prospects were very poor.

But in one respect at least, Mr Y's luck had changed for the better. He was adamant that he wished to die at home – or, at least, that he wished to go through the process of living his last days there. He would consider admission to a hospice but only, ideally, in order to die. The hospital he was in was taking part in a pilot End of Life programme, working to help patients fulfil their wish in terms of place of death.

The rationale for my Primary Care Trust's involvement was clear. Even twenty-four-hour care at home would cost them less than frequent hospital admissions. The hurdles, of course, were significant: Mr Y had no family to look after him, and no savings to pay for private services. Even if the NHS could provide carers, the language barriers would be considerable; there was certainly no local pool of Vietnamese-speaking home helps, and translator services were hard to come by. The tumour was aggressive and, with his death likely to occur within three months, there was limited time to set up foolproof twenty-four-hour-a-day arrangements for his care.

The team on the programme rose to the challenge. The local palliative care nurse took on the task of fast-tracking funding for his care package, and the district nurse joined the meetings held to make sure that every eventuality was catered for before he was discharged from hospital. It was inevitable that acute problems would arise, and we needed to ensure they did not turn into crises. Both the day and night district nursing teams were briefed, and the local Social Services department was recruited to set up a care package through an independent agency. The local interpreter service was paid a retainer fee to offer twenty-four-hour access to translation. And then Mr Y went home.

Fortunately, Mr Y lived in an area which had access to 'hospice at home' services. It is not yet available throughout the country, but it is spreading, and offers twenty-four-hour expertise and support to healthcare staff and families. The government's commitment in July 2008 to extend this sort of service to patients nationwide will help thousands of people for whom the headlines went in one ear and out the other. In this complicated case, the nurses and doctors were more in need of moral support to deal with their anxieties than was the patient.

For almost three months, Mr Y lived successfully at home. He was being visited three times a day by carers, and twice a day by the district nurses, but he began to fear for his ability to cope in the hours between these visits. His anxiety grew as he contemplated the thought of an emergency hospital admission if his condition deteriorated. Then someone told him that the hospice had two Vietnamese cleaners who were prepared to translate for him. That was enough: he agreed to move in. He was too weak to speak for long, but the cleaners spent hours sitting with him – sometimes talking, sometimes just being there. Two days later, in the calm of the hospice, he breathed his peaceful last.

There is nothing which at once affects a man so much and so little as his own death.

Samuel Butler

Be Prepared

The Gold Standards Framework may be spreading fast, but we're still a long way from the day when all of us can take for granted this sort of care. For one thing, getting involved in it is voluntary – which means that take-up is likely to vary across the country. It's difficult to say for certain which parts of the country are doing best: there aren't any nationwide records of how many GP practices are trying to offer this service for all their patients. What's more, there's still a postcode lottery as far as the other services, like twenty-four-hour-a-day nursing or respite care, are concerned.

After eighteen years as a GP, I took six months off to concentrate on the care of dying patients in my area of London. As part of that process, I spent some time at the hospice to which I refer all my palliative care patients. Every morning we had a ward round at which we would discuss each patient. If someone was being considered for discharge home, the first question that had to be dealt with was where they lived. If they came from one London suburb, they could get twenty-four-hour nursing care only if they were deemed to have less than two weeks to live. If they lived just a mile down the road, they could have round-the-clock nursing care however long they had left, but only if the alternative was keeping them in the hospice or sending them to hospital. The permutations, it seemed, were endless. So, it goes without saying, was the bureaucracy.

The government has promised that, within the next few years, everyone in the UK who is near the end of life will have access to all the services they need to die at home, if that is what they want. I first saw this grand aim mooted in a government White Paper in 2003, and dismissed it as yet another cheap attempt at vote-winning. I have been forced to eat my words because the politicians are putting their money (or, rather, our money) where their rhetoric is. Every Primary Care Trust has been ordered to set up a working group to establish what services are needed in its particular area.

When I was first invited to join our local group, I was tempted to refuse on the grounds that this would be another GOBSAT – Good Old Boys Sat Around Talking, reinventing the wheel and never getting anything concrete done. Six months on, I became convinced that this 'bottom up' approach makes sense: each area does have different needs, whether it's because of the racial mix, the average age or the geographical peculiarities of the patch. If you live in an area within half a mile of the nearest twenty-four-hour chemist, for instance, it would be daft not to make use of their facilities. If, on the other hand, the nearest pharmacy – let alone the nearest hospice – is ten miles away down a single-lane track, investing money in having a car stocked with every medicine you might need is right at the top of your agenda.

Once the group has come up with a list of objectives, the government is providing ring-fenced money to put their plans into action. Some of the objectives set by the government are compulsory for every area, although each group can decide how best to implement them. For instance:

- carers and relatives will be guaranteed facilities to stay with their loved one in hospital if they want to
- patients and carers will have access to dedicated telephone advice twenty-four hours a day
- anyone at the end of life will be able to bypass the usual bureaucracy and get access to homecare services if they want to die at home
- local end-of-life coordination centres will allow 'joined up care', unhindered by geographical barriers.

So yes, we're getting there – but slowly. In the meantime, there are lots of ways we could all stack the odds of a good death in our favour. Yet on the whole, we aren't using them. Why not? It could be simply because the lawyers got their hands on them before we did – with the result that they have the most pompous and off-putting titles imaginable. Whoever thought it could be a good idea to replace the self-explanatory term Living Will with the indigestible Advanced Decision obviously needs to get a life. You'd have thought that telling the people caring for you what matters to you, and asking them to take your priorities into account, was simple common sense. But no, we have to call it a 'Statement of Wishes and Preferences'. And to top it all, we have the Lasting Power of Attorney. But more of that later.

Some of these changes may not have been taken up on a large scale because they've only just been introduced. The Lasting Power of Attorney, for instance, became law only in October 2007. Before that the closest we had was an Enduring Power of Attorney (yes, they are fundamentally different), which you could use to ensure that someone you trusted had the power to make decisions for you about your 'goods and chattels', but not about your health.

It seems bizarre to me that for twenty years, ever since the Court of Protection was set up to supervise the implementation of Enduring Powers of Attorney, it has been legal for you to nominate someone to pay your bills, draw your pension, sell your home or put you into care; yet even if you trusted him implicitly, there was no way that you could give permission for your husband to decide if you were to be resuscitated or put on a ventilator. It's only since October 2007, when the Mental Capacity Act (and with it the Lasting Power of Attorney) came into force, that we've had that choice.

Mrs G could certainly have done with a Lasting Power of Attorney. She had cancer of the bowel, which had spread throughout her body. She also happened to have diabetes, which she had always managed well herself, testing her blood sugar regularly at home with tiny blood samples gained by pricking her finger. Because she had type 2 diabetes, and therefore didn't need insulin injections, this monitoring wasn't strictly necessary – but she said it gave her peace of mind to know her blood sugar level. She was a lady who liked to know where she stood. When she was diagnosed with inoperable cancer, she announced that this was obviously why God had given her diabetes in the first place – at least she was used to needles.

Mrs G had been widowed for several years, and lived alone in a one-bedroom flat in sheltered accommodation. She had faced the issues surrounding her death with pragmatic good humour, discussing the possibilities first with her GP and palliative care nurse, and then with her family. Her two daughters were both married with jobs, but their own offspring were old enough to be independent. So the daughters arranged to stay with her every night and weekend and, when the time came, they would take leave from work to care for her at home.

The district nurses were visiting regularly and continued to check her blood sugar. There was absolutely no need for that: even a lethally high level of blood sugar would probably have offered a relatively peaceful demise. The only treatment is intensive, involving admission to hospital, intravenous drips and hourly blood tests. It was not an option if she wanted to stay at home to die. But details are easily forgotten, and somehow the regular testing was never cancelled.

Over the next few weeks, Mrs G's condition weakened and she became more and more drowsy, although she was not distressed. The tumour had spread to her brain, and time was short. Her family prepared themselves for a peaceful goodbye at home. But they reckoned without her blood results. Her blood sugar became higher and higher – possibly because of the tumour in her brain. The district nurses rang the hospice, who recommended more frequent visits to check on her, but no treatment since she was so peaceful.

The consultant from the hospice spoke to Mrs G's daughters on the phone, reassuring them and trying to prepare them for the very end. Two hours later, their mother was not opening her eyes, and one of the daughters rang the hospice again. She had been told that this situation was likely, but was still desperate to know if there was anything else she could do. In her anxiety she rang the wrong number, and got no reply. Panicking, she rang 999, and within minutes an ambulance was at the door.

Seeing an unconscious patient with a list of ever-rising blood sugars, the ambulance crew felt they had no choice but to admit Mrs G to hospital – and it was here that it all went wrong. Not because she was denied treatment – her medical management was 'by the book' for a patient in a diabetic coma – but because the doctors on call were adept at saving lives, not losing them.

The daughters' first action was to inform the doctor that their mother was terminally ill. His response? 'That may be, but that's not what's killing her. I can't allow someone to die from a treatable condition – that wouldn't be ethical.'

So Mrs G was 'saved' from her diabetic coma with intravenous drips and blood tests, including regular samples taken from the arteries deep in her groins, to check the level of oxygen in her system. As her blood sugars came down she roused herself, plucking at the drips in her arms and pulling away from the blood tests. By the time her blood sugar was normal three days later, she was only semi-conscious because of the tumours in her brain.

The Welcome Visitor

At her daughters' insistence she was sent home, where she died two days later without regaining consciousness. She had her peaceful end, but she was totally unaware of it. Her last conscious moments were spent fighting alien needles in a hostile, unfamiliar hospital ward. Despite all our planning, her last days were exactly what she had tried so hard to avoid – and all because the hospital doctor insisted on saving her life.

At the opposite end of the spectrum, Miss J used the Lasting Power of Attorney to ensure that her death progressed exactly as her life had done – in just the way she planned. Fifteen years ago, she had breezed into my consulting room with a copy of her Living Will. To say that I was taken aback was an understatement – not only was this the first example of a Living Will I had ever been asked to file in a patient's notes, but she was a sixty-year-old in rude health who lived alone and worked as a legal secretary. She immediately began to interrogate me on my knowledge of the legal status of Living Wills (basic in the extreme), asking how I could guarantee that the hospital would be informed immediately by me of the existence of the will if she were admitted unconscious (I couldn't, unless she was admitted by me or one of my partners) demanding details of the surgery's system for ensuring that original copies were kept safe in the event of fire (non-existent).

Be Prepared

If I have painted a picture of a deeply scary lady, that's because she was – at least to me, and at least then. I had been a partner for only three years and was still facing new challenges on a daily basis. Here was a representative of the legal profession (bound to sue me) who had uncovered my inadequacies (it was bound to happen some time, but I'd fooled all my patients so far) within minutes of our first encounter.

Over the years that followed we developed an understanding and, I hope, a mutual respect. Frighteningly intelligent and fiercely independent, Miss J possessed a brusque manner which hid a mass of insecurities. She had never married, and harboured a secret fear of dying alone with nobody caring enough even to notice her absence. Even worse, she had an abiding terror of being helpless and was anxious to prevent any doctor being able to condemn her to a living death as a 'vegetable' (her word) because of a well-meaning determination to pull out all the stops, regardless of the likely outcome.

On 1 October 2007 she was back in the surgery. With a matter-of-fact air she pulled from her capacious handbag a sheaf of papers, which she deposited on my desk. This, she announced, was her Advanced Decision. After four years spent researching for this book, I should have remembered that this was the new name for what used to be called a Living Will. But the new regulations had only been in place for nine hours, and I had morning surgery, not legal niceties, on my mind. My confusion must have been obvious because she sighed and put on the familiar, patronising voice that over the years must have caused her employers to check that their ties were straight and their nails clean.

Hadn't I seen any other patients yet this morning? she asked. Had nobody but her understood how momentous today was? Today was the day 'they' (those unnamed doctors who might be called upon to care for her in an emergency) stopped having any choice. Finally, her Living Will had legal status, meaning that 'they' had no choice but to abide by it.

With exaggerated patience, she opened the official-looking document and started to take me through it. I did not have to ask Miss J if she was sure she'd fulfilled all the requirements, and I meekly settled down for a refresher course in the small print.

In this, as in so much else, the meticulous Miss J was right – an Advanced Decision does indeed now have legal status, but only if it's written in a specific way:

- It must be signed, dated and witnessed
- If you want your Advanced Decision to include refusal of life-saving treatment, you have to record

explicitly that your decision stands 'even if life is at risk'

- You need to make it clear that you're 'of sound mind', and that you know the Advanced Decision will only 'kick in' when you're incapable of making your wishes known

- It applies only to treatment you want to refuse: being put on a ventilator; being tube-fed if you're in a coma etc. You can't specify what you *do* want, such as: 'If I have breast cancer and I'm unconscious because it's spread to my brain, I still want to be given Herceptin.' (Needless to say, Miss J had that side of things covered, too – but more of that in a minute.)

- And now for the really tricky bit. Unless you're absolutely determined that you don't want to have a particular treatment – say, cardiac resuscitation – under any circumstances, you have to be very specific. It's not good enough to include a blanket clause such as 'I don't want to have cardiac resuscitation if the chances of success are small.' After all, for one person a one-in-five success rate might seem miraculous, while another might see it as an 80 per cent chance of failure. Miss J's list included the following:
  ◦ If I am terminally ill and expected to die from my underlying condition within the next three months, I do not wish to be treated with

antibiotics if I develop pneumonia or to be resuscitated if my heart or breathing stop
- If I am unable to swallow, I do not wish to be fed by a gastric tube
- If I suffer a stroke which affects my level of consciousness, I do not wish to be resuscitated.

Miss J had also brought with her a separate Statement of Wishes and Preferences about things she did want. Unlike an Advanced Decision, a Statement of Wishes and Preferences is not legally binding, and you can't over-ride the doctor's judgement of what is in 'your best interests'. For instance, you can't insist on being put on a life support system indefinitely if you're in a car crash and are brain-dead when you arrive at hospital. The good news is that you don't have to get your Statement of Wishes witnessed, or even write your wishes down. In fact, as part of the Gold Standards Framework doctors and nurses involved in end-of-life care already use them widely. You can also include non-medical wishes, such as religious or spiritual preferences. What's more, the team looking after you have to take your wishes into account, which in practice means they will usually accommodate them if they possibly can.

Miss J's Statement of Wishes and Preferences was short, but very much to the point. Regardless of her level of consciousness, she wanted to be on a single-sex ward; she wanted to have her torso, front and back, covered at all times when she was not actually being examined or washed; she wanted to be washed or toileted only by female staff; and she wanted every member of staff to introduce themselves to her when they met her for the first time. She also wanted to have the reason for any medical procedure performed on her explained to her, even if she was classified as unconscious at the time.

As she read out the last wish on her list, she smiled almost mischievously. In bold print she had typed across the bottom of the page, 'I wish to be left entirely alone by any spiritual advisor of any persuasion.'

Left alone? I queried.

'Well,' she explained, 'the Advanced Decision only lets me refuse medical treatments. The Statement of Wishes and Preferences includes non-medical areas, but it only lets me specify what I do want, not what I don't. I lost any faith I might have had a long time ago, and if this is the only way I can stop the so-and-sos from getting me when I'm vulnerable, that's what I'll do.'

Miss J had also presented me with a copy of her Lasting Power of Attorney, giving her nephew the power to make decisions about her treatment if she was not able to do so. Given how detailed her Advanced Decision was, I expressed my surprise that there might be any eventuality she had not anticipated. 'Belt and braces, my girl' she smiled, patting my hand. 'You can't be too careful. I'm not going to risk going in to bat without someone to fight my corner.' I tried to ignore the image of her in a boxing ring, cricket bat in one hand and boxing glove in the other.

I had met her nephew before. A thin, bespectacled and rather earnest young man, at first he had struck me as rather too meek to 'bat' on anyone's behalf. But that was before we moved on to the subject of the right to die. He suddenly came to life, arguing as passionately as his aunt about the right of the individual. She had chosen her champion well.

Every Lasting Power of Attorney has to be lodged with the Office of the Public Guardian before it takes legal effect. Somehow, I was not surprised to hear that she had made her appointment with them in person later that very day. She could have posted it to them. The new Office had only opened that day and I knew that teething problems were likely. She would probably end up waiting for hours before some young bureaucrat informed her pompously that she did not need to deliver the forms in person. I almost felt sorry for them.

In the end Miss J needed her braces as well as her belt. Six months later, she suffered a massive stroke. This left her with a rare condition called 'locked in syndrome': she could understand, but could not communicate, move or even swallow. It was the same condition that the journalist Jean-Dominique Bauby chronicles so movingly in his book, *The Diving Bell and the Butterfly*. In his case, it took months for the staff looking after him to teach him to communicate by blinking his left eyelid: the only movement he had control over. He dictated his memoir with painful slowness, each letter spelled out with blinks.

Miss J had no intention of living long enough to dictate anything but the plans she had came close to being derailed. She had collapsed on holiday, and the doctors had put in a gastric tube to feed her before they knew of her wishes. As soon as her nephew arrived he made them aware of her wishes in no uncertain terms. Under the terms of her Advanced Decision, they had not just the right but the duty to remove the gastric tube. But there were procedures to be followed first and procedures take time.

In the meantime, she developed pneumonia. One of the over-enthusiastic doctors at the hospital pointed out that under the terms of her Advanced Decision, she was theoretically not 'terminally ill': many people who have strokes live for years. As far as he was concerned, then, he should treat her infection with antibiotics.

Miss J's nephew was having none of this. Once the tube to feed her was removed, she would slowly starve to death but because of the stroke, she would be conscious. Pneumonia was her chance for a relatively quick end and he meant to let her take it. Three days later she was gone.

Considering that all men are mortal, we are curiously unwilling to acknowledge that death, our inevitable fate, should not always be postponed.

Baroness Warnock
When to Die (published 2006)

I I

Killing from Kindness

Advanced Decisions can only be a good thing. They offer reassurance to the patient, and make life easier for the doctor when it comes to crucial decisions. The final years of my father's life could have been so different if they had been available to him. When I first wrote about his death in 2003 I said that the doctor caring for him had increased his dose of morphine until it killed him. I said the same about the death of my former wife, and I based those comments on what I was told at the time by nurses and doctors. They assured me that they would never allow a patient to suffer, and increasing the morphine dose to a fatal level was an accepted procedure. That seemed to me to be eminently sensible and humane. So I was both puzzled and upset when I received letters from several doctors – including experienced consultants – challenging what I had written. One consultant told me that he had worked in three hospice units and two cancer centres and with three Macmillan community teams – and had never seen it done.

So what is going on here?

The answer lies in something called the Doctrine of Double Effect. Most of us have never heard of it and there is no reason why we should have done. What it means is that a doctor can give a patient drugs that may kill him – but only so long as he is doing it to relieve that patient's pain. That seems pretty straightforward. It's not. It's an ethical quagmire.

The strongest painkillers we have in this country are called the opioids, which include morphine and diamorphine, otherwise known as heroin. It is impossible to read a newspaper or watch a television crime programme without being aware that an overdose of heroin can kill you. It happens tragically often. But in the right dose, opioids are often the only way of controlling the pain of someone who is in the last stages of illness. About four out of five people dying in hospices are given morphine in the last few days of their lives.

How our bodies react to a drug depends on all sorts of things: our age; our weight; any other drugs we might be taking at the time. Our pain threshold is another important factor. If we have a low threshold of pain it's obvious that we will need a bigger dose than if we have a high one. So pain relief always involves a certain amount of trial and error. A sensible doctor will start with the minimum dose and increase it gradually until the pain is gone.

So far, so good. It involves no ethical issues – just

sensible treatment. The problems arise when the pain is so great that a massive dose is needed – one that is likely to stop the patient breathing. The doctor knows that if he continues to increase the dose the patient will die. To put it more bluntly: the doctor will have killed the patient.

The most recent studies suggest that this does not happen often, but it is impossible to put even a roughly accurate figure on it for obvious reasons. When people are in the terminal stages of a terrible illness such as liver cancer they will die whatever the doctor does. Sometimes the doctor genuinely will not know whether it was the diamorphine or the illness that stopped the heart. So the doubt is always there. Short of rewinding time and giving the patient exactly the same treatment without the morphine, the doctor cannot possibly be certain which one caused death. What many believe is that without the medicine the patient would not have had a longer life in any meaningful sense of the word – just the wretched prospect of a longer death. Hence the Doctrine of Double Effect.

It says to the doctor: It is possible that you may kill a patient, but if you have done so in the process of trying to relieve suffering you cannot be held to account. That, you might think, is all the reassurance a doctor needs to do what he believes is in the best interests of the patient. Not so. As one put it, the great fear for a doctor who is trying to relieve the patient's pain is not that he might kill him by accident. It is that those left behind will believe that he killed him on purpose.

This is more than paranoia on the part of doctors. Even though they can call on the Doctrine of Double Effect to justify their actions, there is always the fear that they might possibly be charged with manslaughter or even murder. It has happened several times in recent decades.

The first time the doctrine was invoked in a British court was in 1957, in what newspaper headlines at the time described as the murder trial of the century. The GP in the dock was the infamous John Bodkin Adams, who had given such a massive dose of painkillers to an elderly patient that she died. Mr Justice Devlin – later to become Lord Devlin, one of the most famous judges of his generation – pronounced that a doctor is entitled to 'relieve pain even if the measure he took might incidentally shorten life by hours or perhaps longer'. Adams was acquitted.

It was an extraordinary verdict, not just because that particular patient had left Adams £157,000 in her will – a massive sum at the time – but because no fewer than 160 of his patients had died under suspicious circumstances. In a subsequent trial Adams was found guilty of thirteen offences of prescription fraud, lying on cremation forms, obstructing a police search and failing to keep a dangerous drugs register. But he was never convicted of murder. He was removed from the Medical Register in 1957 but reinstated in 1961. The Doctrine of Double Effect had been established.

Some forty years later a Northumberland GP, David Moor, was charged with murder after he had given diamorphine to a terminally ill patient. What made his case different was that he had agreed to be interviewed by the *Sunday Times*. The interview was published the day after the patient died, and in it Dr Moor admitted that he had given many of his patients diamorphine to help them have a pain-free death. The case went to court and the doctor was acquitted.

When Lord Joffe, an advocate of assisted dying, was giving evidence to the House of Lords about the need to change the present law, he highlighted the anxiety that doctors face. It is clear, he said, 'that there are a number of doctors who are concerned about using the double-effect principle in order to ease the pain of their patients because they are frightened that they may be prosecuted'. Sarah knows exactly how they feel.

I only knew Mr V for a single day – but in that day I watched his wife go through a lifetime's-worth of emotions. One Sunday in late autumn I was on duty for my west London practice when I received a call about a terminally ill patient I had never met. I had been a GP for only two years, and my experience of terminal care was limited.

Mr V and his wife lived in a flat in a large, rambling house. They had met in their mid-forties, each with a failed marriage behind them.

Setting themselves up here, in an area populated with many nationalities, colours and creeds, was an adventure – their first home together, and a completely new start. They built their married relationship among the colourful sari shops and wandered for hours around the ethnic food emporia, expanding their culinary repertoire. Every restaurant held romantic memories for them.

When they first arrived, the estate agent's optimistic take on the area was 'colourful'. Run-down and sometimes downright dangerous was probably nearer the mark. They set about transforming their home, with a jaunty brass doorknocker and hanging baskets of flowers at the entrance. Over the next few years, more and more of the houses in the area were transformed back into their former pastel-painted glory, complete with English Heritage interiors. Wine bars and bistros replaced the late-night corner shops, and taxis door to door were no longer a matter of self-preservation as soon as darkness had fallen.

During their life together they travelled widely. Neither had children, and they revelled in the opportunity to explore Sumatra, Tanzania, Laos and the Philippines together. Their bookshelves were lined with lovingly labelled photograph albums documenting each step of their shared voyage through middle age.

Ten weeks earlier, at the age of fifty-eight, Mr V had been diagnosed with pancreatic cancer. He had felt off colour for weeks, but had convinced himself that he was simply overworked and in need of a break. By the time he went to his GP, he had lost half a stone in weight and was barely able to walk to the shops. Cancer was a prime suspect.

Survival rates for pancreatic cancer are among the worst in the large and varied cancer family, but Mr V's decline was even faster than most. Although he had met the Macmillan nurses, he hadn't had a chance to make any preparations to die at home. But this, his wife assured me, was the one thing of which he had been absolutely certain.

When I met Mr V he was bedbound, drifting in and out of consciousness and unable to speak. His distress and pain, however, were all too clear. His bed had been moved into the sitting room, which led straight off the tiny front hall. His wife's body language, when she first answered the door to me, seemed confrontational and almost aggressive – yet as I watched the softening of her expression as she set eyes on her husband, and the infinite tenderness with which she wiped his forehead, it was clear that there was more fear than anger. She was terrified at the thought that I might deprive her of the right to fulfil her last promise to her husband – to care for him to the end in his own home. Here was a woman struggling to hold herself together.

Much later that day, I learned why Mrs V had been so suspicious – she had seen her father admitted to hospital as her mother stood timidly by. He had wanted to die at home, but his wife had panicked and called an ambulance. Once he was in the Accident and Emergency department, she asked to take him home. But by then it was too late. The doctor had advised her mother that she 'wouldn't cope right at the end all on your own with him dying in front of you'. Mother and daughter had seen him die a lingering death in an open ward, surrounded by medical paraphernalia. And Mrs V was terrified that, like her mother's, her courage to see her husband's life right to the end would fail in the face of a nameless doctor's disdain.

As I examined her husband, I steeled myself to find the right words to communicate how serious her husband's condition was. Until the day before, his pain had been controlled with liquid painkilling medicine – but since then he had been unable to take so much as a sip for many hours. I knew he would need a pump to release a slow stream of diamorphine directly into his system. I also knew that she would realise this was the beginning of the end, and that I would have to break the news. The prospect was terrifying. Although I had explained the practicalities of a loved one's final hours as a junior doctor in hospital, I had never done so in someone's home. In the hospital there were nurses on hand to offer tea and comfort, or a medical superior to advise on the most appropriate words to use. This was different.

Yet again – for the thousandth time since I had left the protection of my GP training posts and qualified as an 'independent practitioner' – the reality of the seemingly innocuous term 'independent' hit me. It felt like the wrong word: I was totally alone and utterly isolated. 'Independent' was getting my ears pierced without asking my parents' permission. 'Independent' was moving away from home into my first student rooms, but with parents only a phone call away to offer advice on the right temperature to wash colour-fast cotton or how to fit an electric plug. 'Independent' was dealing with my first cardiac arrest, or my first solo forceps delivery of a wrinkled baby into its proud father's arms.

As well as explaining to Mrs V exactly what her husband needed, I had to make it happen. Hospice services have progressed at a breathtaking rate in recent years, but out-of-hours services have not. I knew I could access the medicine through the on-duty pharmacist, but the equipment to get it into Mr V's system was another matter entirely. We may only have heard about the 'postcode lottery' in the

NHS over the last few years, yet as far as access to emergency medical equipment was concerned the postcode lottery was, even in the early 1990s, very much alive and kicking.

I left Mrs V and drove back to the surgery to get hold of the phone numbers which I hoped would lead me to an immediately available pump. As I drove, I tried to rehearse the words I would use to Mrs V. GPs spend years honing their consultation skills, learning to adapt their language and approach to what they know about the person they are dealing with. But I did not know Mrs V at all, and I was about to give her the worst news of her life. Each explanation sounded more brutal, more hopeless, than the last. Did Mrs V have any idea that one of the side-effects of diamorphine was to interfere with the patient's ability to breathe? Did she realise that while we could try to control his pain before we reached this dangerous dose, there was a chance that we would not? Would I for ever be to her that woman who turned up and promptly killed her husband? When he died (which he would) would she blame me, or even claim that I had killed her husband deliberately?

In the event, that first discussion was not as awkward as I had feared. Mrs V was only too aware of how distressed her husband was, and distraught that she had not been able to help him. When I promised that both the medicine and the pump would be there within the hour we became partners in his care, not adversaries.

The nurse duly arrived and I assembled the pump. She was comforting and eminently competent, radiating the confidence that comes with twenty years' experience. I only wished that the same could be said of me, because I was the one who had to decide how much medicine to give. I started timidly, with a hopelessly ineffectual dose. This was serious, grown-up medicine and I had never coped with anything remotely similar on my own.

Mrs V had been holding herself together – just – since I had made my suggestion about relieving his pain. As the seconds ticked by, and his inarticulate moans failed to diminish, it was to me that she looked imploringly for help. Never before had I felt such a fraud – and never had it been more important that I hide my own insecurity.

I explained that I had tried a small dose in case Mr V was particularly sensitive to the effects of the medicine, and that there was much more we could do. Ever since I have lived with the knowledge that, if I had been braver with the dose, I could have relieved his suffering more quickly. Today, no doctor qualifies as a GP without knowing all about the twenty-four-hour advice service from the hospice. But in the early 1990s training for terminal care was in its infancy. I had never been inside the local hospice and I had no idea I could turn to my colleagues for help.

I left several times when I was called to visit other patients, but returned after each visit – as much for my sake as for Mrs V's. I spent more time talking with Mrs V that day than I usually do with a patient in the course of a year. We spent our time in the sitting room next to her husband's bed, both aware of every change in his breathing. As the hours passed, and Mrs V shared with me more details of their life and travels together, I was left in the surreal position of getting to know a man whose physical form lay on the bed beside me – almost a ghost between us.

Mr and Mrs V not only had no children, but no close relatives either. Their best friends were away, and Mrs V could not bring herself to telephone anyone less intimate and ask them to come and support her. It was just the two – or, rather, the three – of us.

After about the fifth increase of dose had failed to provide relief, I decided that the time had come to broach the subject of side-effects. Or, as I did not say in so many words, I had to make her realise that the dose he needed to control his pain might be only slightly less than a dose that would kill him. My own adrenaline levels were so high that I can't remember a word of how I phrased it but the relief I felt at sharing my concern was enormous. I do remember that Mrs V smiled at me sadly when I finished and thanked me for my honesty. I understood then that the same thought had occurred to her, and that we had both been trying to pluck up our courage to put our thoughts into words.

I adjusted the dial on the pump with far less trepidation than I had on the previous occasions – and almost immediately Mr V stopped breathing. I came perilously close to panicking: could I have killed him that fast? Had I made the wrong adjustment? But as I stared at his wife's frozen expression Mr V took another gasping intake of breath, and within a few minutes he was breathing more calmly. We had found the right dose to ease his distress at last.

Three hours later, without stirring again, Mr V finally stopped breathing. Mrs V sat completely still beside him, his frail hand softly clasped between hers, her breathing rate unconsciously matching his. For about ten minutes after he died she sat completely still, then brushed his hair out of his eyes and kissed his eyelids. Then she looked up, gazing at me intently. 'You really don't have to be upset,' she said. 'You know it wasn't you who killed him.'

Come lovely and soothing death,
Undulate round the world, serenely
    arriving, arriving,
In the day, in the night, to all, to each
Sooner or later, delicate death.
                                        Walt Whitman

12

Taking Control

From everything Sarah has written in the past few chapters it is clear that doctors are increasingly aware of their obligation to help their patients achieve a good death as well as a longer, healthier life. But it is equally clear that they will not always succeed – either because of the nature of the final illness or because of human nature. We are all different and we all react to serious illness in different ways. Some of us can cope reasonably well and some of us cannot. Some of us display extraordinary fortitude and want to fight to the bitter end; some of us choose simply to give up and turn our faces to the wall. Some of us – for whatever reason – believe fate should take its course; some of us want to seize control and end our lives in the way we think best. Some of us regard life as a sacred gift and the very notion of suicide as repugnant; some of us believe that if monotheistic religions such as Christianity place freedom of will at the heart of their doctrine, then we are entitled to choose how we end our lives in just the same way as we choose how to live them.

We have moved a long way from the days when the body of someone who had committed suicide was dragged through the streets, face down, before being hung from a gibbet or thrown on a rubbish heap. That was what Louis XIV decreed should happen in France in the seventeenth century. Attempted suicide is still a crime in some countries. It is punishable by up to a year in prison in India and Singapore, for instance. But in most countries suicide is no longer illegal – which is progress of a sort. It was always preposterous in any secular state that attempted suicide should have been a criminal offence.

Laws that cannot be enforced make idiots of the lawmakers. It is one thing for a religious believer to be deterred from suicide by the prospect of spending eternity in hell – or even being buried beyond the walls of the cemetery – but quite another to threaten someone who is genuinely prepared to contemplate suicide with the might of the law. How, in the name of logic, do you punish someone who has managed to kill himself?

The notion of suicide as a crime ended in continental Europe in the wake of the French Revolution, when the idea took root that if there were no king and no established religion there could be nobody against whom it could be a criminal act. In Britain the famous English jurist Sir William Blackstone pronounced in his *Commentaries on the*

Laws of England that suicide was a crime against the monarch, who was the head of the established Church. It remained a crime right up until 1961 when the law was changed – and it changed in a most peculiar way. It was no longer a crime to kill yourself, but it became a crime to give help to someone who wanted to do precisely that. In other words, it is now illegal to help someone do something that is itself legal. The maximum penalty is fourteen years in jail.

The sad reality is that there are many people who want to end their lives for reasons most of us may be able to understand and sympathise with, but who are not – for one reason or another – capable of doing so. They need help. In a perfect world the help would consist of persuading them that their life really is worth living – perhaps by reassuring them that it is possible to relieve their pain when it becomes intolerable. But this is not a perfect world. There are some diseases so hideous and unrelenting that, even with the best treatment, the final days or weeks or even months will be more than some people can bear. Or perhaps I should say: more than they believe they will be able to bear; it amounts to the same thing. The fear of pain can be greater than the reality. They want to know – more than that, they *need* to know – that they have the option of ending their lives before that point is reached.

There are others who do not have a terminal illness but have, perhaps, been horribly disabled by illness or accident and cannot face the rest of their lives imprisoned in their own bodies, unable to do anything for themselves. Some are able to overcome the obstacle of their useless bodies with sheer will and mental determination. The great physicist Stephen Hawking is an awe-inspiring example of that. Some simply have the dogged determination to make the best of what fate has bequeathed them. Others give up and want nothing but release from their private hell. They present any civilised society with some of its most profound moral questions, and I shall be addressing them in Chapter 13.

In a practical sense, this subject has taken on much greater urgency over the past few decades – partly because of the medical advances that Sarah has written about in earlier chapters. We have choices now that we did not have a generation or two ago, when the diagnosis often amounted to an early death sentence. The longer doctors are able to keep us alive, the more people there will be who may decide they prefer the alternative – people who don't want to be kept alive.

Another important factor is the huge amount of publicity given to the growing number of people who choose to end their lives at a death clinic in Switzerland. What was unthinkable has become not just thinkable but do-able. Euthanasia and assisted suicide are in the news and on the political agenda as never before.

So let's look first at how it works in those countries where people are allowed to get help to end their lives. That help differs from country to country. It may be a form of euthanasia, where a doctor carries out the final act, or it may be assisted suicide, where the doctor gives the patient the necessary drugs. In almost every case the basic requirement is evidence of free will on the part of the person who wants to die – though, as we shall see, even that can be something of a grey area. The various systems differ as to whether the patient must be terminally ill to 'qualify', whether they might recover, whether they are in great pain, and their state of mind.

In fact, surprisingly few countries have any legislation in this area – which may be partly thanks to the barbarity of the Nazis in Germany. In the late 1930s they launched, in secret, a programme of 'involuntary euthanasia' codenamed Action T4. A simpler codename for it would have been murder. They started out by killing children under the age of three who were severely disabled mentally or physically, and then extended it to older children and adults who were deemed to be living a 'life unworthy of life'. It was to be a couple of decades before the euthanasia societies that had begun to form in the United States and some European countries were able to resume their campaigning.

Then, on 29 March 1974, a twenty-one-year-old woman, Karen Ann Quinlan, went to a party near her home in the United States. She drank far too much and took too many drugs, and when she came home she collapsed. Twice she stopped breathing for at least fifteen minutes. By the time she was admitted to hospital she had lapsed into what doctors today call a persistent vegetative state. Day after agonising day her parents sat at her bedside watching their beloved daughter as her body wasted away and a machine did her breathing for her. Her only movement was the occasional uncontrollable thrashing of her limbs.

After several months they accepted that they had lost their daughter. In truth, as far as they were concerned they had lost her on 29 March. But she was not at peace. So they asked the doctors to turn off the machines that were keeping Karen Ann alive. The hospital refused. Her parents went to court and won. Two years after that drunken party, the respirator was switched off. But instead of dying, Karen Ann was able to breathe for herself. Her parents might have hoped that this would be one of those 'miraculous' recoveries that are occasionally reported, when someone who has been in a coma for years suddenly 'comes alive' again. But the reports can be cruelly misleading: it does not happen when the brain has been damaged as badly as Karen Ann's had been. Breathing was all she could do. Nothing else. For nine long years she lay in her hospital bed, her parents praying that her suffering would come to an end. Eventually it did. She developed complications from a bout of pneumonia, and in 1985 she died.

Her short life and lingering death had a profound influence on public opinion in the United States, and eventually on the medical profession. Millions were moved by her story and wondered why Karen Ann and her parents had had to suffer so much for so long. One practical outcome of the Quinlans' legal battle was the creation of formal ethics committees in hospitals, hospices and nursing homes, and there was also an acceptance of living wills in some states. But above all, it helped establish the legal precedent that doctors should be allowed to end treatment that was keeping a person alive if all hope of recovery had long since vanished. And it ignited a passionate debate across the nation between those who held that life is sacred and only God can determine when we die, and those who held that no one should be condemned to suffer unnecessarily.

Another nine years were to pass after the death of Karen Ann Quinlan before any significant legal changes were introduced in the United States. In 1994 physician-assisted suicide became legal. Politicians approved a law that allowed doctors to prescribe lethal drugs to terminally ill people who wanted to die – but only in the liberal state of Oregon and only for people who were judged to be in the last six months of life. The Oregon law was to become the model pursued by campaigners for assisted suicide in other American states and countries – including Britain – who were impressed by the conditions laid down. In 2006 the US Supreme Court – the ultimate legal authority in the land – upheld the Oregon law. Two years later the people of Washington State voted for something almost identical. Other states are thinking of doing the same. These are the main safeguards:

- The patient is given a prescription rather than the medicine itself and has to take it to the pharmacy to get it made up. Then it must be drunk at home. If the patient is incapable of swallowing it, he cannot be helped to do so by his doctor and the doctor cannot administer an injection.
- Two doctors have to confirm that the patient has less than six months to live. This is meant to guard against 'slippery slope' worries – specifically the fear that unscrupulous relatives might take matters into their own hands or doctors might come to regard themselves as gods and simply dispense with people they think no longer have any value for society.

- The patient must have made two written requests, at least fifteen days apart. This provides a cooling-off period.
- The requests must be signed by two witnesses, one of whom is not related to the patient. This guards against relatives pressurising them into asking to die for financial reasons.
- Two doctors must have confirmed that the patient is mentally capable of making the decision, and does not have a mental health problem (including depression) which might affect their judgement.
- The doctor must discuss all the alternatives with the patient, including hospice care and pain control. This is to make sure that they really have considered all the alternatives.
- The doctor has to encourage the patient to let their next of kin know about their decision.
- They can change their minds at any time.

There is one other condition. Anyone wanting help with killing themselves must live in Oregon and must have known their doctor for some time. This is designed to stop something that's become known rather gruesomely as death tourism. It happens in Switzerland, the first country in Europe to allow any form of assisted suicide.

It goes back to 1918, when the Swiss were developing a national penal code. They decided that because suicide was not a crime, helping someone to die could not be a crime either – within certain limits. It would depend on the motives of the person doing the helping. When a law was finally introduced in 1942 it made it a crime if the helper stood to benefit in any way or had put any pressure on the person who said he wanted to die. What the law did not do was demand that there should be an established relationship between the person who wanted to die and the person helping them.

The result of that, for people who were desperate to get help with killing themselves and could not get that help at home, was predictable. Switzerland became the place to go, even though for some years the only place in Switzerland that catered for the 'death tourist' was the Dignitas clinic in Zurich. Since it set up shop in 1998 it's believed that more than a hundred people have gone there to die from Britain alone, though it's impossible to verify the figures for fairly obvious reasons.

The word 'clinic' creates a rather misleading impression. It was opened, not in a pristine hospital building with white walls and shiny equipment, but in a residential apartment building in a city suburb. Because it was on the fourth floor the only way to remove the bodies from the building was in the lift. Unsurprisingly, the residents were not too happy to be sharing the lift almost every day with a body bag. One former resident was quoted in the *British Medical Journal* as saying, 'I used to get panic attacks as I was confronted with death every day. Sometimes you would meet the people in the hallway before they went upstairs, and a short while later their body would be carried out. I had to endure it for a year before my contract on the flat ran out.'

Now the 'clinic' has been moved to an industrial estate on the outskirts of the city. It was there that a British doctor, Anne Turner, went to die. Dr Turner was about as far removed from the lovelorn teenager playing at suicide to draw attention to herself as it is possible to imagine. She was a GP in her mid-sixties when she developed a progressive and incurable degenerative disease called supranuclear palsy – the same disease that killed the brilliant musician, comedian and actor Dudley Moore. Dr Turner knew exactly what to expect – not only because of her considerable medical knowledge but because she had seen her husband, also a GP, die of a similar disease a few years earlier. She knew that it would rob her of every movement, including the ability to speak or even swallow. Eventually she would be unable to breathe and she would die. The death would be prolonged and slow, and she would lose every vestige of her independence and dignity. She preferred to die before that happened. So she tried to kill herself. She used sleeping pills, anti-depressants and a plastic bag, but she failed.

At every attempt she was brought back to life by well-meaning people who believed they were acting in her best interests.

So she decided to go to the Dignitas clinic. She told her family what she intended to do. Her children were, unsurprisingly, shocked and tried to talk her out of it, but her mind was made up and in the end they went to Switzerland with her. So did a BBC film crew and reporter whom she invited to join her. Dr Turner wanted the world to see what she was doing and why.

Shortly before she boarded the plane in January 2006 she said, 'I saw what happened to my husband, and I don't want to end up like that, and I don't want to end up like Dudley Moore, who could not walk, talk or even blink.' The pictures of Dr Turner setting off for Switzerland were profoundly moving. They showed a woman, surrounded by her loving family, who appeared to have so much to live for and yet was setting out on what every viewer knew would be the last journey she would ever make. Although she needed a walking stick in order to get about, in every other respect she seemed as fit and lively as many another sixty-six-year-old. She smiled and joked, and exhibited not an ounce of self-pity. There were two things that made her angry, though: the fact that 'people talk to me as though I am stupid' and the fact that she had to travel to a foreign country to do what she had desperately wanted to do at home.

She felt that she had been robbed of life – a curious thought from someone who had decided to kill herself – but in one important sense she was right. What she was most terrified of was that she might leave it too late, and the disease might have reached the stage where she would have been unable to travel. Then the slow death she so feared would have been inevitable. So she was forced to err on the side of caution and make the journey while she was still fit enough.

'I am not looking forward to it,' she said, 'but at the same time I am. I had this awful fall last night and could not get up. I thought then that this really demonstrates that what I am going to do is right.'

On arrival in Zurich she went straight to the Dignitas clinic, where she was asked if she was acting under any form of duress. She said she was not. She was given the drugs she wanted, and a few hours after arriving in Switzerland, she was dead.

Less than three years later another Dignitas 'patient' from Britain hit the headlines in a far more dramatic fashion. Craig Ewart was an American university lecturer who had moved to Britain to teach at Edinburgh University. In June 2006 he was told that he had motor neurone disease. Soon afterwards he decided, like so many others, that he would end his life in Switzerland. What makes his story unique is that he and his wife, Mary, agreed to allow a documentary film to be made of his final months.

Professor Ewart became the first person to be shown ending his life as the camera rolled, and millions of television viewers watched him breathe his last.

The programme, shown on Sky television, triggered a storm of controversy. Mrs Ewart, who was at her husband's bedside, was entirely unrepentant. 'It was what we both wanted,' she said, 'and if this film gets people thinking about death and talking about it, that's all that Craig would have wished.'

That's exactly what Dr Turner wanted too. They wanted to put an end to what they called the taboo surrounding suicide. This was one of Dr Turner's last comments: 'Doctors should be able to help people to die. I had a cat, and I had him put down because he was riddled with cancer, but we cannot do that with humans.'

No, we cannot 'do that' with humans – neither in Switzerland nor anywhere else for that matter. The cat cannot ask to die and that, as Dr Turner well knew, is the crucial difference. You cannot help someone die if it is not utterly clear that they want to be helped – however pure the motive, however much you might want to end that person's suffering. To do so would be involuntary euthanasia at best and manslaughter at worst. That would clearly be illegal – although in some cases the rules are applied in such a relaxed fashion that the boundaries seem to have become dangerously eroded.

It might be helpful to define what we mean when we talk about euthanasia. The Oxford English Dictionary has this simple definition: 'the means of procuring a quiet and easy death'. The organisation Care Not Killing (CNK), which is an alliance of organisations opposed to it, defines it thus: 'the intentional killing by act or omission of a person whose life is felt not to be worth living'. It outlines three different kinds of euthanasia:

Voluntary – where a mentally competent patient requests it

Involuntary – where a competent patient is not consulted

Non-voluntary – where the patient is not competent to make the request

It becomes more complicated when a distinction is made between so-called 'active' and 'passive' euthanasia. Active means, in essence, administering an injection, and passive means withholding treatment or withdrawing it.

In Belgium a Euthanasia Act was passed in 2002. It stipulates that it must be the doctor who administers the lethal dose. In other words, voluntary euthanasia is legal but assisted suicide is not. The patient has to make more than one request to the doctor, and the procedure cannot be carried out until at least a month after a request has been made in writing. The patient must be 'in a futile medical condition of constant and unbearable physical or mental suffering that cannot be alleviated'.

So those are three different countries with three different versions of mercy killing. And there is a fourth partner in this *dance macabre*: Holland, whose laws are probably the most liberal of all. Under the old legislation it had been illegal to perform euthanasia or help people kill themselves. A number of doctors were prosecuted, but convictions were rare and punishments negligible. It was clear that public opinion was in favour of a change in the law and in 2002 it happened. From then on a doctor who performed voluntary euthanasia or helped someone commit suicide was no longer criminally liable.

The biggest and, for many people, most worrying difference between the Dutch and some other systems is that it is possible for people who are not in the final stages of a terminal illness to be helped to die. Instead, their condition must be 'lasting and unbearable with no other reasonable alternative'. But there have even been some cases where patients have been helped to die by their doctors because they are 'tired of life'. There are other significant differences. It is possible for someone to make a Living Will (an 'advanced statement') in which they ask for physician-assisted suicide as opposed to simply asking that their treatment be discontinued. It is also possible for children as young as twelve to request and receive help to die.

In many other countries – including Britain – various laws have been considered and either rejected out of hand or put in the pending tray. In Chapter 13 I shall be looking at the moral arguments.

Death is not anything ... death is not ...
It's the absence of presence, nothing more
... the endless time of never coming back
... a gap you can't see and, when the wind
blows through it, it makes no sound.

Tom Stoppard

13

The Doctor's Dilemma

The interesting thing about ethical and moral debates is that the more complex they are, the simpler they sometimes appear to be – depending on where you started out. Abortion is a pretty good example of that. It's always wrong in the eyes of the so-called 'pro-lifers' (I've always wondered if there is anyone out there who is actually 'anti'-life) because they believe life begins at conception. Full stop. If you are approaching it from the opposing position it is equally simple: a woman has an inalienable right to choose what she does with her own body. Full stop again.

The question of assisted suicide and euthanasia is arguably even more complex and ethically fraught than abortion but, once again, you'd never think so if you listen to the fundamentalists. This is roughly how it goes:

'Killing is wrong, isn't it?'

'Yes, of course it is. But is it still wrong if someone wants to be killed?'

'Yes.'

'Why?'

'Because life is sacred. God gives us life, and only God can take it away.'

Thus, for many, the debate begins and ends with the sanctity of life. It's wrong to kill, and that's that. So let us try this little ethical dilemma, which is often presented to young doctors by ethics professors who want to challenge their preconceptions about what the 'sanctity' of life means in the real world of impossibly difficult choices.

A New York patrolman responds to an emergency on the highway. A truck has crashed at high speed, smashing into the concrete pillar of a bridge which has partly collapsed on to his cab. The driver is trapped. His legs are crushed in a tangled mess of twisted metal under a massive concrete block. The only way to get him out would be first to drag the concrete block off the cab and then cut away the metal. It would need heavy lifting equipment and hours of work with oxy-acetylene burners. But the truck is carrying a load of highly flammable liquid which has caught fire and is beginning to turn the cab into a furnace. The driver knows he cannot possibly be rescued before he is burnt to death. He screams at the policeman, 'Please shoot me now!'

That was the dilemma Sarah and her fellow medical students were presented with on the first day of their course on medical ethics. The professor made it clear – as all good ethicists would – that there are seldom absolute rights and wrongs. But he invited any student who believed that the policeman would be wrong to kill the truck driver to leave the course there and then. He was not being arrogant or dismissive of their beliefs. He was not saying, 'If you had been in that position and refused to put the driver out of his agony you would necessarily be a bad doctor.' Instead he was saying, 'If you believe so utterly in the sanctity of life that you would never, even under the most extreme circumstances imaginable, consider ending it, then there is no point in continuing with this course because nothing I can do could persuade you otherwise. The rest of the course would be completely irrelevant.' All the young doctors stayed for the rest of the course.

The policeman's dilemma is crucial in the debate about mercy killing because it demonstrates – admittedly in a rather melodramatic fashion – that the sanctity of life cannot be the beginning and end of the argument. Could anyone with a shred of mercy in their soul have refused to put that imaginary truck driver out of his agony? How could the policeman have stood there and watched him being burnt to death? He could not. So the real point of the dilemma is that it establishes the principle that there are circumstances in which we would be prepared to end someone's life prematurely if we found ourselves in a position to do so.

Doctors, obviously, find themselves in that position more than anyone else, but it's seldom (if ever) as clear-cut as the policeman's dilemma. It is not only about ethics; it's about the law too. In the United Kingdom it says they must allow someone to die if the person is a mentally competent, mature adult and has made a clear request to end the treatment. Ideally the patient will have already done so with an Advanced Decision. What the patient cannot do is ask the doctor to take active measures to put an end to their life. The doctor cannot inject or proffer the poison. It becomes much more difficult if the patient is not a competent adult, but a small child – perhaps a newborn baby. So let us put the drama of the burning truck to one side and move into the relative calm of one of our large teaching hospitals.

My own wife Edna – about whose death I wrote earlier – had worked in a teaching hospital in Cardiff. When she finished her training in the 1960s and qualified as a staff nurse she opted to work on a special unit – the first of its kind in the country – dedicated to the care of babies born with spina bifida. It was a particularly demanding job for any young woman who loved children. It could be immensely rewarding, but it could also be heartbreaking.

Given the right treatment, many of the babies would eventually be able to lead full lives, but some were born so hideously deformed that the only humane approach was to allow them to die. With some pretty heroic surgery, it might have been possible to keep them alive for a while, but the outcome would never have been in question. So, instead, they were allowed to slip away quickly and quietly. Edna often wept for them, but she never doubted that she and her colleagues were doing the right thing. I sometimes wonder how she would have reacted if I had accused her all those years ago of mercy killing, but I think I know what she would have said: it would have been wrong to raise the hopes of the parents and prolong the suffering of the child.

But forty years ago medicine was so much less sophisticated and our expectations of what it could achieve so much lower. The relationship between doctor and patient was different, too. The presumption was almost always that the doctor knew best, and we tended not to challenge medical opinions in the way we do today. There was still a vestige of unthinking deference lingering in those post-war years, and anyway we had no internet to turn to for an instant second or third opinion. So, in most respects, life was much less complicated for the average doctor. It simply did not occur to Edna or to me, come to that, to question what happened on her unit. It was simply accepted as the way things worked. It would not be accepted today, and nor should it be. It was wrong for the medical staff to be expected to play God and exclude the parents. The final decision as to how those pathetic babies were treated or not treated might rest with the doctor, but the parents clearly had the right to be consulted.

Medical ethics is quite clear on the subject. A competent adult has a right to refuse treatment, even it means they die. A parent has a right to make a similar decision on behalf of their child, as long as the child's doctors agree that they are acting in the child's best interests. The problems start if the doctors believe that what the parents decide is not in the best interests of the child. In that event, the doctors have a right to apply for a court order to force the parents to agree to treatment.

In fact, it works both ways. If doctors and parents disagree, the courts can be asked to step in, regardless of which party thinks treatment should be withheld. In the 2000s we have seen parents going to court to force their child's doctors to continue treatment, even though the doctors thought the baby's quality of life was so poor that he or she should be allowed to die peacefully if the heart stopped again. And in November 2008 a thirteen-year-old girl's parents were threatened with a High Court order when they supported their daughter's decision to refuse a heart transplant. In the event, the child protection officer who met Hannah quickly judged her competent to make the decision for herself, and she was allowed home to die in peace.

The euthanasia debate today enters different territory. Let's leave the spina bifida unit of forty years ago and move to another part of the hospital where older babies are treated. Imagine a scenario in which a doctor is talking to the parents of a one-year-old boy (it's mostly boys who are affected) who has what is known as Hurler's syndrome. The doctor is a specialist in the disease and knows exactly what it will do to the child. His joints and bones will seize up. He will suffer terrible pain and will be shunted in and out of hospital for countless operations. His brain will not develop normally, so it will be impossible for him to understand why he is being put through all this misery. His eyesight may well fail. He will be dead by the time he is fourteen – perhaps sooner – and he will probably have spent as much time in hospital as he will have spent at home. He will have had a wretched life and his loving parents will have suffered with him. Should he be killed?

We hardly need to ask the question. Even if the parents suggested it and the doctor privately sympathised with them, he would have to refuse. The law as it stands would leave him with no option. Yet, on the face of it, there are half a dozen powerful reasons for ending that little boy's life.

So many people would be spared so much suffering over the years to come. The child himself. His parents. Any other children they may have, whose own young lives would be blighted by the effect of a desperately ill sibling on both them and their parents. The NHS would save a fortune on the cost of all those operations and hospital treatments – money that could be spent on curing people who have a real hope of recovering.

We can all probably add to that list. But still the answer would be no. Surely no civilised society would even contemplate the premeditated killing of a sick child. That's the kind of thing the Nazis did. But note that word 'society'.

What if the doctor or the nurses, who had watched other children with the same condition die slow and painful deaths, felt deep in their hearts that it would be cruel and inhumane to allow this child to suffer in the same way? And what if the parents agreed? What if they decided among themselves that a quiet, painless overdose, slipped in through one of the many needles and drips protruding from the baby's delicate little frame, would save him from years of suffering?

No questions would have been raised beyond that hospital ward because no one else need have been involved or need ever to have known what had happened. No courts. No official inquiries. No ethics committees. No newspaper headlines or columnists passionately debating the pros and cons. No questions in Parliament. No politicians or prelates pontificating on the *Today* programme. Just one more tragic death of a child born without hope. One small child at peace, his parents free to devote their lives to caring for their other children.

The parents and the medical staff would have acted out of love and compassion – just as my late wife did on her spina bifida unit and just as the fictional New York police officer would have done had he aimed his pistol at the truck driver's heart and pulled the trigger. And, in my view, they would have been wrong.

Moral dilemmas really do not get more difficult than this but in the end it must be for society as a whole to resolve them. Individuals, however much they may have the interest of the child at heart, cannot take it upon themselves to decide the fate of another human being who is unable to make the decision for himself. A small child is, by definition, unable to do so. Agonising though they may be, cases such as this must be tested in the court of public opinion.

One difficulty with any form of mercy killing is always going to be reconciling the collective interest – the interest of society or the community – with that of the individual.

Primitive societies had no such problem. In some ancient civilisations a newborn baby might be removed from its mother and left out on a rock, exposed to the elements, for twenty-four hours. Those that survived were the strong ones.

They would thrive and, as they grew older, the community would be strengthened. Those that did not would probably have died early anyway (or so it was assumed), and attention and scarce resources that could have been better used elsewhere would have been wasted. It was undeniably brutal, but what mattered above all else was the survival of the group – scarcely different, in its practical outcome, from the way a very old elephant will wander off to die rather than stay with the herd and weaken it.

We may, in these more enlightened times, recoil from such barbarity but it had an unmistakeable logic: the interests of the individual are often over-ridden by the interests of the community.

That, of course, was one of the arguments that Stalinists used in order to justify the vile police state in the old Soviet Union. The interests of society always took precedence over those of the individual. So what if a hundred innocent men and women were tortured and murdered by the fearsome security apparatus – or even a million? One of them just might have been a subversive who could have threatened the regime. That was all the justification they needed.

One of the great moral principles that civilised societies have come to accept and enforce over the centuries is that a country or regime should be judged by the way it treats the most vulnerable members of society. Sometimes that principle is over-ridden – in time of war, for instance, when bombs are dropped on a city centre. Then, the slaughter of civilians is justified on the basis that national survival is at stake. But that is a hideous aberration. For generations, in Britain at least, we have been struggling to create a more tolerant, decent society. We have abolished slavery, created a welfare state and a National Health Service, ended the persecution of homosexuals and women who need an abortion, criminalised the ugliest forms of racism. In every case we have recognised that minorities, the weakest and poorest and least advantaged, need the protection of society as a whole. I would argue that few people are more vulnerable than those who are denied the right to end their lives in a manner of their own choosing.

The organisation Care Not Killing (CNK) believes it is a mistake to see the legalisation of physician-assisted suicide solely in terms of individual rights and to ignore the impact of such a radical change in the law on society. If doctors are asked to help kill people, they say, that would of necessity damage the relationship between them and the community they serve. Such suicide would 'acquire an aura of clinical respectability'. It seems that many doctors in the United Kingdom – perhaps most – share that view. Here is what the General Medical Council had to say in 2005: 'A change in the law to allow physician-assisted suicide would have profound implications for the role and responsibilities of doctors and their relationships with patients. Acting with the primary intention to hasten a patient's death would be difficult to reconcile with the medical ethical principles of beneficence and non-maleficence.' Yet there is no evidence from countries where physician-assisted suicide is legal that the relationship between doctor and patient has been damaged.

The CNK makes the perfectly sensible point that most of us assume the advice we get from our doctors will be in our best interest, but it goes further with this claim:

> It is but a short step from there to the notion that, if my doctor is prepared to prescribe a lethal overdose for me, he must regard that as an appropriate form of treatment for my medical condition and he must feel that taking my own life is preferable for me as a patient to dying naturally. In other words, physician-assisted suicide is being placed within the comfort zone of a social service (the healthcare system) which patients trust and which they assume, rightly under the legal status quo in Britain, is geared to protecting their interests.

Is it really a 'short step' from acceptance of the principle to a doctor regarding mercy killing as preferable to a natural death? I doubt it. What worries the anti-euthanasia lobby is that the relationship between a patient and a doctor will end up being no different from the relationship between a customer and a supplier in any commercial market. The patient who wants to die might say, 'This is what I demand, and if you won't supply it I shall go elsewhere.' Making it legal for a doctor to help a patient die would, they argue, represent a significant step towards the principle of the patient calling the tune.

Yet why not? Why should they not call the tune, assuming that the patient is an adult who knows what he is doing and is neither under pressure nor mentally incapable?

Of course the practice of medicine is different from selling houses or cars. There will be – there must be – times when the doctor refuses a patient what he or she wants. It's a pity, for instance, that more doctors don't refuse antibiotics to patients who demand them when they have a nasty case of the sniffles. Giving in to their demands will do the patient no good (colds are caused by a virus, and antibiotics have no effect on viruses) and will harm the wider community because of growing resistance to antibiotics. And there will be times when the doctor will try to insist on a particular course of treatment that the patient does not want. But there's a pretty basic point here: each of us owns our body and each of us is, ultimately, responsible for our own destiny.

That crucial fact has been recognised time and again by legislatures around the world who have legalised abortion. If a woman can decide to end the life of an embryo that might conceivably survive outside the womb, on what basis can we claim that she does not have autonomy over the means of her own death? However much I respect my own GP (and I respect her a great deal), in the end I want to be able to make that final decision for myself. And so, if opinion surveys are any guide, do most people. The most recent UK polls show that about 80 per cent of us are in favour of some form of mercy killing. That obviously leaves a sizeable minority who are not – and it is a highly influential minority which includes the Church of England, the Roman Catholic Church, Orthodox Jews and pressure groups such as Care Not Killing. Recent history suggests that those who are opposed to mercy killing are more effective in their opposition than those who are in favour. Religious passions run high on this. As for politicians, they tend to be rather more scared of a well-organised, angry minority than of a relatively moderate majority.

For many politicians this is one of those highly controversial issues where it is much easier to take cover in the grey area. Mercy killing already happens, so why invite trouble by legalising it? There's some strength to that argument. As we have noted time and again in this book, doctors not only allow people to die when it would be possible to keep them alive a little longer, they even deliberately hasten their deaths. What is not generally known is how often it happens.

Professor Emily Jackson of the London School of Economics is regarded as one of Britain's leading authorities on euthanasia. She makes the point that in palliative care it is routine to administer doses of analgesic drugs which are 'virtually certain' to bring about the patient's death. Another factor is the 'DNR' order, which is regularly included in patients' medical notes. DNR – as every nurse knows – means 'Do not resuscitate.'

Professor Jackson asks this crucial question: 'A doctor who withdraws life support will usually simply be doing her job, whereas a doctor who gives a patient a lethal injection might be found guilty of murder and receive a mandatory life sentence. Given that the intention and the outcome in each case might be indistinguishable, what justification can there be for endorsing the former while treating the latter as a crime of exceptional gravity?'

The answer, she suggests, is that it makes sense only if we ignore the perspective of the individual patient and look at it purely through the eyes of doctors. That might have been regarded as ethically acceptable until the 1960s, but since then medical law and ethics have increasingly focused on the patient's own perspective. In relation to euthanasia the current legal position 'necessitates a peculiar and wilful disregard for the individual patient's point of view'.

Perhaps the most common attack deployed against legalising any form of mercy killing is the 'slippery slope' argument. Where will it end? Once we embark on this road surely there is a danger that people who are going through a bad patch in their lives, feeling depressed, unable to see any point in living, will call at the doctor's surgery one grey February morning and demand help with putting an end to it all. Many of them, the argument goes, would live to regret it – if they lived – but they have the law on their side and they know their rights.

It's an alarming prospect, given how many people contemplate suicide at some time in their lives. But it's absurd to suggest that anything like that is likely to happen in a properly regulated system. The law would not allow it. There would be too many safeguards built in, and doctors would be only too aware of them.

Ah ... the doctors. We trust them, don't we? Well, yes, opinion polls show that they are still widely respected and more trusted than any of the other professions. But aren't we asking them to do something they are sworn not to do, and is there not a huge danger in giving them a legal power over life and death? Surely there is a risk that too many doctors will become accustomed to playing God and knocking off patients right, left and centre when they decide that their lives are no longer worth living? Or even when the patient becomes too much of a nuisance?

And since we are taking such a bleak view of human nature, let us consider this from the viewpoint of the rapacious relatives too. There is nothing more upsetting, they might feel, than a very old granny who clearly has nothing to live for except making everyone else's life a misery. It's even worse if she is in poor health and makes incessant demands on the family as, regrettably, so many do. It's worse still if the young family is desperately struggling to make ends meet and Granny has a nice big house she doesn't need and a tidy little sum tucked away in her bank account and she simply refuses to die even though she's had a really good innings. Selfish, eh? At this rate the family will never get their hands on her wealth. Naturally, no one would dream of doing anything about it. You cannot go around knocking off old grannies, can you, however persistently they cling on to life? But maybe applying a little pressure to make her realise what a burden she has become might not be a bad idea... .

Naturally, good people like you and me would never dream of allowing such unworthy thoughts even to cross our minds, but that word 'burden' is a hugely emotive one in this debate. Baroness

Warnock, a philosopher who has become highly influential in the fields of education and medical ethics, used it when she spoke to a journalist from a Church of Scotland magazine in the summer of 2008. Here is part of what she said: 'I am absolutely fully in agreement with the argument that if pain is insufferable, then someone should be given help to die. But I feel there is a wider argument that if somebody absolutely desperately wants to die because they are a burden to their family or the state, then I think they too should be allowed to die.' Clever though Lady Warnock undoubtedly is, she is likely to have damaged her cause with that comment. It would have helped reinforce the sceptics' view that this is dangerous territory: encouraging people to feel they almost have a duty to put an end to their lives if, say, they become demented. It might even, the sceptic would argue, allow relatives to apply pressure to them to do the decent thing and put an end to their 'useless' lives.

It is impossible to prove that none of this will happen. There are some bad people out there, and they will sometimes do bad things. Harold Shipman literally got away with murder for many years when he was, on the face of it, a caring family doctor. But if we followed the slippery slope logic to its ultimate conclusion we would never do anything. It has been used by opponents of all kinds of human endeavour over the years – especially pioneering research in the field of human reproduction – and there are millions of happy families in the world today who would not exist if it were not for the development of IVF.

There is an even more powerful argument against the slippery slopers, based on the old saw that there's no need to use a crystal ball when you can read the book. It's called experience.

Until a few decades ago we had no way of knowing for sure how doctors and their patients might react to new laws. We do now, because we can look at what has happened in other countries where they have been introduced.

The model that appeals to campaigners for mercy killing in the United Kingdom is the one I described in Chapter 12 that was adopted by Oregon in the 1990s and has since been adopted by Washington State.

It appears that most people in Oregon know about the law, and many have considered using it. About one in six dying patients talk to their relatives about the possibility and about one in ten of those have looked into the question of whether they were 'eligible'. Of those who went as far as asking their doctor for a prescription, only about one in ten actually took it to the pharmacist to have it made up. According to research published in the *New England Journal of Medicine*, between 1998 and 2007 physicians wrote a total of 541 such prescriptions and 341 people died as a result of them. About 86 per cent of those who took the drugs were in hospices, and 81.5 per cent had terminal cancers.

As for those who asked for prescriptions but never took them to the pharmacist, it seems that what they wanted was an 'insurance policy' in case their suffering became too great and they could not face the prospect of going on any longer. According to some of the doctors involved, many people find it reassuring to know they have a choice, even though only a tiny minority actually take that final step. So, in the ten years after physician-assisted suicide was introduced in Oregon, it was used by fewer than forty people a year out of a population of nearly 4 million. That figure has remained constant.

The final argument deployed against any form of euthanasia or assisted suicide is that if the present system ain't broke, why fix it? The problem here is that there are an awful lot of people who believe it *is* broke, and a smaller number who have suffered and are still suffering as a result of it. In one six-week period in Britain there were three different cases involving people who wanted to end their lives but needed help to do so. The system had let them down.

Dan James was a promising young rugby forward – good enough to play for England as a teenager and with every chance of a successful professional career.

Nicknamed 'Cowboy' by his friends for his tough, rugged appearance, he had a boisterous approach to life and was full of energy and ambition. In 2007 – four days after he had helped England Students beat a French team – he turned up for a training session at Nuneaton RFC in Warwickshire. What happened that afternoon destroyed his life.

Dan was practising a scrum manoeuvre when the pack went crashing down – hardly an unusual event, but this time he ended up at the bottom of the heap and was crushed under the weight of several beefy young men. Bones in his neck and his spinal column were dislocated. In the weeks to come he had several operations and spent eight months in rehabilitation, including a stay at the famous Stoke Mandeville hospital. But none of it worked. He was able to move his fingers – and that was all.

Those who knew Dan said he was an intelligent young man, strong-willed and determined. He simply could not face spending the rest of his life helpless in a wheelchair. He was incontinent, suffered uncontrollable spasms in his legs and upper body, and needed care twenty-four hours a day. Over the months that followed he tried to kill himself and failed. After the third attempt he begged his parents to help him die and in the end they agreed that they would take him to Switzerland. In September 2008 his life ended, as so many others have done, in the Dignitas clinic outside Zurich.

If the ultimate tragedy for any parent is to lose a child, how much greater is the anguish of knowing you must spend the rest of your life remembering that you were instrumental in bringing it about. But for Mr and Mrs James, there seemed no alternative. Here's how Dan's mother expressed it: 'What right does any human being have to tell any other that they have to live a life filled with terror, discomfort and indignity? What right does one person who chooses to live with a particular illness or disability have to tell another that they have to?'

But that is not how the law sees it. When Mr and Mrs James returned from Switzerland they discovered that a woman who worked for their local social services had called the police. They were questioned by officers and, in the days and weeks when all they wanted to do was mourn their son, they had to endure the agony of worrying that they would be charged with aiding and abetting a suicide, for which the maximum sentence is fourteen years in jail.

'I hope', said Mrs James, 'that one day I will get the chance to talk to this lady... Our son could not have been more loved and, had he felt he could live his life this way, he would have been loved just the same. But this was his right as a human being. Nobody, but nobody, should judge him or anyone else.'

In the event, they were not charged. Keir Starmer, the Director of Public Prosecutions, ruled that even though there was sufficient evidence to take action, a prosecution would not be in the public interest. Far from encouraging their son to kill himself, he said, the couple had tried to talk him out of it. He added, 'Daniel, as a fiercely independent young man, was not influenced by his parents to take his own life and the evidence indicates he did so despite their imploring him not to.'

This was an enormously significant announcement, not so much because of the decision (none of the British 'accomplices' in Dignitas suicides has ever been charged) but because of the way in which Mr Starmer announced it. It appeared that he was effectively ruling out even the possibility of future prosecutions in similar circumstances. Yet the law does not allow him to do that. It is perfectly clear: it is illegal to 'aid, counsel or procure the suicide of another'. Mr Starmer said – he had to say – that his decision was based on the 'very specific and unique' facts of the James case.

This is, as many jurists concede, an almighty muddle. How can it be anything other than aiding and procuring if someone makes all the arrangements for a suicide, buys the tickets, pays the fees of the clinic and physically enables the sick person to make a journey they would have been incapable of making by themselves? That is why Debbie Purdy – someone else who feared she would not be able to have the death she wanted – went to court.

When Ms Purdy was diagnosed with progressive multiple sclerosis in 2001 at the age of forty-five she knew it was a death sentence. The only question was how long she would take to die and how painful and undignified it would be. Like so many others with terminal and crippling diseases she wanted to die at home – with the help of her much-loved husband Omar – while she still had some semblance of control over her life and before the suffering overwhelmed her. She knew that the law in Britain would make that impossible, so she felt her only option was to make the trip to Switzerland.

Again, she would need Omar's help. She could not do it without him. But what if a zealous prosecutor in Britain decided to make an example of him and dragged him into court? It might even mean that he would end up in prison. That was a risk he was prepared to take out of his love for her but, out of her love for him, it was not something she would allow. And so, in June 2008, she appealed for a High Court review of the law on assisted suicide on the grounds that the Director of Public Prosecutions had acted illegally by not providing guidance. She wanted a ruling that would answer a simple but vital question: would Omar, and others in his position, be prosecuted on their return to this country or would they not?

She knew the stakes were high because the court, backed into a corner and forced to reach a decision,

might rule in favour of prosecution. But if Debbie
Purdy's body was weak and failing, her spirit was
strong and determined. She was fighting not just for
her own right to die in the way she chose, but for
the many others who would surely follow her. She
made a powerful plea to the court. Here's part of
it:

> My dearest wish would be to die with dignity
> in my own home, with my husband and other
> loved ones around me. I hate the idea of having
> to travel to another country when I will be at my
> weakest and most vulnerable, both emotionally
> and physically.
>
> Going to another country also means that I have
> to go earlier, because being able to travel such a
> distance and to make all the arrangements in a
> foreign country will require me to be physically
> and mentally capable. That, too, will mean that
> my life is further shortened as a result of the lack
> of a humane law in this country. I hope that one
> day the law will recognise that this is inhumane
> and that the law should be changed.

On 29 October 2008 the High Court delivered its
ruling. Debbie Purdy had won the 'great sympathy'
of the judges but she had lost her case. Lord Justice
Scott Baker said, 'This would involve a change in
the law. The offence of suicide is very widely drawn

to cover all manner of different circumstances; only Parliament can change it.'

The last attempt to change it in Parliament was in 2006, when the human rights lawyer Lord Joffe introduced the Assisted Dying for the Terminally Ill Bill in the House of Lords. It was based on the Oregon system, which is regarded as having more safeguards built into it than in any other in the world. Joffe's bill had even more.

The patient would have to make a written request to his doctor for assistance and a consultation with two doctors, one of whom would have to be an independent consultant. If either had any worries about the patient's mental competence the case would have to be referred to a psychiatrist. There would then have to be a minimum period of fourteen days for reflection, and the patient would also have to consult a specialist in palliative care. Only after all this could a final, written request be made to a doctor for a prescription, and it would have to be the patient, not the doctor, who administered the drugs.

But Lord Joffe QC came up against Lord Carlile QC, and in the battle of the two barrister barons it was Carlile who was to triumph. Joffe claimed that because Carlile opposed his bill at the second reading it meant there could not be a full debate and the details of the bill could not be properly examined. It was, he said, a serious break with parliamentary tradition. Carlile responded by saying he had done so because this was no run-of-the-mill private member's bill but one that contained life-or-death proposals involving serious issues of principle. Either way, the bill was defeated and that, as things stand, is that. Joffe says he will try again one day, and in the meantime the battle of the barristers continues. They are no longer fighting in the chamber of the House of Lords, but in the columns and letters pages of the newspapers.

Wherever it happens, it must be right that we continue this debate. The Prime Minister Gordon Brown has made his own position clear. In December 2008 he told MPs he would never support legislation to permit assisted suicide that might put sick or elderly people under pressure to end their lives. Some politicians criticised him for breaching a convention that says governments should not express views on matters of conscience rather than party policy, but in a democracy such as ours the best place to have this debate is on the floor of the House of Commons.

As I write, there are moves in Scotland to bring in a law there that would allow assisted suicide. If that were to happen it would put even more pressure on politicians south of the border. It's one thing for people to travel to Switzerland to die; it would be even more bizarre if they merely had to drive north a few miles from Newcastle.

As I have tried to show, the present system is not working. It did not work for my father in the closing years of his life, nor for young Dan in his youth. It is not working for Debbie Purdy who, as I write, faces the prospect of making that dreadful one-way journey to Switzerland and the fear that she will leave her beloved husband to face the possibility, however remote, of a criminal trial.

Yet still the opponents of euthanasia say it is right to deny them the last of life's great decisions – the ability to choose how they leave this world.

In this chapter I have tried to balance the rights of the individual against the greater good of society. I have viewed it from the perspective of those vulnerable people who want to be helped to die in a way they believe will minimise their suffering and allow them to go with dignity. But there is a final argument from the anti-euthanasia lobby and it is, on the face of it, a powerful one. It is about palliative care.

CNK claims that those countries which have legalised assisted dying have relatively poor records in this field. Britain, by contrast, is a world leader; palliative care has been a recognised clinical speciality (like, for example, oncology or paediatrics) since 1987. We have, as well as many hospices for in-patients and out-patients, specialist palliative care departments in most major hospitals. Physician-assisted suicide, it says, would risk undermining all this. It is the need to go the extra mile in relieving intractable symptoms that has led to some of the most significant breakthroughs in palliative medicine. Assisted suicide would 'provide a bolthole for lazy doctors'.

Well, would it? That is the question Dr Sarah Jarvis will address in Chapter 14.

Life itself is but the shadow of death and souls departed but the shadow of the living.

Sir Thomas Browne

14

Who Decides?

It's both tempting and comforting to believe that we doctors know what we are doing, and usually we do. It's not by accident that the death rate from heart disease in the UK has halved in twenty years. Even if I don't know what something is, I can usually say with certainty what it is not. That matters a lot. If a patient comes in with headaches, for instance, my biggest concern is to rule out a brain tumour or meningitis. Once I have done that, where we go next depends largely on the patient and why they have come to see me. If they can cope with the headaches themselves, but not with the anxiety of whether they signal something more sinister, I can reassure them and leave it at that. If they need a precise diagnosis because the headaches are causing them to stop functioning, we would take a different tack. We would look in more detail for the cause, even if it didn't change the outcome.

So on the whole I am used to knowing the answers to the important, life-threatening questions. But as far as perhaps the most important question of all is concerned, I often don't have a clue. That question is: '*When* am I going to die?'

Knowing the answer to the question: '*Am* I going to die?' is often the easy bit. In the long term, the glib answer is, 'Yes, we all are sooner or later.' In the short term, doctors can often give patients an idea of the likelihood by using statistics based on thousands of people's experience. Depending on the type and stage of your cancer when you are diagnosed, your chance of surviving could be as high as 95 per cent; or the only question might be when, not if.

But one thing we cannot tell you with any degree of certainty is when you are going to die. For instance, it never crossed my mind that my mother would die within three weeks of being diagnosed. Statistically, it should have been more like three months. But my mother, like my patients, was more than – and more unpredictable than – a statistic. And the uncertainty, the not knowing, is often what distresses my patients most of all.

As time goes on, and more and more people survive into really old age, that question will get harder, not easier, to answer. With terminal cancer, doctors can usually be accurate about how long a patient has left to within weeks, or at least months. With heart failure, and even more with dementia and frailty, the answer to the question: 'How long have I got?' is: 'How long is a piece of string?' The statistics tell me that Mrs M, with her failing heart and kidneys, should have breathed her last a year ago. In fact, she is going from strength to strength. But for every Mrs M there is someone who has died within weeks, or lingered miserably for months. With dementia, you could succumb to a fall within weeks or decline gradually and inexorably for years.

Much of this change in the length of time people with terminal illnesses stay alive is down to the fact that medicine has advanced in leaps and bounds. And even when we doctors reach the stage where we can't keep you alive for ever, we can at least relieve your suffering.

In fact, one of the most common arguments against assisted dying is that medicine has moved on. It's not that long ago that if you got cancer, you would suffer. If you were lucky, your last days on this earth would be a living hell. If you were less lucky, it would be your last weeks or even months. One way or another you would suffer, because doctors simply didn't know how to relieve the pain, the nausea, the breathlessness.

Now, for most people, we can do precisely that. Many people with cancer do more than avoid a bad death – they die well. It's not just the shift in attitude and the compassion which have come with the development of the hospice movement which have made this sort of good death possible. It's the huge advances in our knowledge of the way the medicines we already have can be used, and in the development of new drugs which can fight these terrible symptoms.

Palliative medicine is advancing every day, conquering new problems one by one. The online community, palliative drugs.com, is an incredibly vibrant and active virtual family, where doctors and nurses all over the world can share solutions to almost every problem which arises. And arise, of course, they do – the human body is adept at inventing new forms of torture.

But these advances have brought new challenges. In fact, so many things have changed in the last few decades that all doctors should re-examine their thinking on the subject. It's not that we have changed our beliefs; it's more that the circumstances have changed. As the economist John Maynard Keynes put it when he was accused of changing his mind; 'When the facts change, I change my mind – what do you do?'

First, we may be able to keep more people alive for longer, but we cannot cure them all. What's more, we cannot always give them the quality of life they find tolerable. We can control symptoms for most – but not for all. In the years to come more and more people will go through a slow decline, gradually losing their dignity but kept alive through the very medical 'advances' we doctors are so proud of.

Second, we doctors have had to enter the real world. When the NHS came into existence half a century ago, the only reason we couldn't cure everything was because the cures had not been invented. While we may still not have all the cures, we have far more than we did, over and above the advances we have made in keeping symptoms under control when the condition is past the stage of cure. The trouble is, in recent years we have been forced to admit that we simply cannot afford to make every new treatment available to everyone who wants it. When I qualified, NICE was an adjective my English teacher disapproved of, not an acronym for the body which decided which treatments I was allowed to prescribe. Even when patients are very much alive, I have had to come to terms with not being able to give them everything.

Third, my patients now see other people in the same position being offered an alternative end to their suffering. When I first qualified, no country in the world sanctioned assisted dying. When it first became legal, it was limited to a few people who lived in the country concerned. Then Dignitas came on the scene. Almost inevitably, the media took a huge interest in Britons going to Switzerland to die, and today scarcely a week goes by without the issue being aired in the press. It is hard for anyone – let alone a dying patient – to miss.

So we doctors can no longer hide behind the fact that assisted dying is only an academic argument. Dignitas has made sure of that. And for some of us, that possibility becomes a reality. And that reality can change our minds.

One of my colleagues, Dr Eric Rose, had always been opposed to the idea of assisted dying. But after a lifetime in practice, a personal experience with just one patient caused him to think again. The patient's name was John Close. Like Dr Anne Turner, Mr Close suffered from motor neurone disease. By the time he saw a news item about Dignitas, he could not stand or swallow and he communicated through a computer because his speech was impossible to understand. A few months later, he travelled to Switzerland to die.

Five years after his patient's death, Eric spoke warmly to me about 'this charming man'. He remembered vividly the day that John came to him to ask for a certificate stating that he was suffering from an incurable condition. Eric knew he would give it to Dignitas. He knew that here was a man who had been given the best medical care possible, but who was still absolutely determined to die. He gave John the certificate, although he admitted that he had grave doubts about whether he would want to be the doctor prescribing, let alone administering, the medication that ended John's life. I struggled a bit with that logic. Eric had issued the letter which John would give to Dignitas but was uncomfortable with the idea of ending someone else's life, no matter how much that person wanted it.

Part of me sympathised with his predicament. I know how anxious I have felt, even when giving a pain-relieving medication, knowing that it might shorten somebody's life by just an hour or two. But I couldn't help feeling that if anyone in society has a duty to come down on one side of the fence or the other, it must be the doctor.

If a doctor believes it is fundamentally, morally wrong, that belief must be respected. Of course nobody should be forced to help a patient die. But if we accept that for some people, sometimes, assisted dying is the only humane option, we have to follow that logic to its natural conclusion.

Doctors have to be involved in assisted dying; he and I are doctors. Would we be happy to do it ourselves? Admittedly he is probably not alone in choosing the middle ground. In Oregon, with its population of 3.7 million, only forty-five doctors issued the eighty-five prescriptions needed for assisted suicide in 2007. But what if those forty-five doctors, too, had decided they approved in principle of assisted suicide but were not prepared to be personally responsible? Where would that leave the patients who wanted (they would say needed) to die?

Like Eric, I spent almost twenty years as a doctor believing that we had moved so far that euthanasia was unnecessary. I really thought that being able to control physical symptoms like pain was enough.

I suppose I was convinced that everyone had the potential to change their mind about wanting to die. Then Mrs W came along.

I had known Mrs W for years. She was a real old-fashioned Londoner who had lived through the Blitz in the Second World War. When her children were small she had stayed at home for thirteen years before returning to work as a nursery nurse. Her husband had been a foreman at the local hospital for thirty-nine years, and she had nursed him for the last six years of his life after he had suffered a stroke. For most of that time she had retained her sense of humour and her cheerful outlook on life, but four months before he died her husband suffered a second stroke, which left him completely helpless. What she found most distressing was that, near the end, his helpless state left him prone to infections which made him confused and aggressive.

She confided to me after his death that those four months had robbed her of her 'proper' memories. Until his second stroke she had still seen him as he was in the early years of their courtship and marriage: kind, funny, charming – in fact her very own Prince Charming. But try as she might after his death, she could not think of him without his irrational outbursts of anger and violence getting in the way. She told me often that she would much rather die than be in that position herself.

Three years later she was admitted with cancer to the local hospice, where she had decided she wanted to die. She was perfectly rational and calm, but kept steering our conversations back to the idea of dying *now*. She had, she told me, done all the important bits of dying: telling her family how much she loved them, and making her peace with God. There was no more reason to stay alive, and every reason to die.

It was not that she worried about the pain: she had been reassured by the staff that they could control that. What worried her was getting confused and saying things she didn't mean to her children and grandchildren. Her grandchildren had been robbed of the chance to remember her husband as the hero he had once been to them. She wanted to die while she was still the sweet doting grandma she wanted them to remember. So as she became weaker, she banned her family from visiting at all just in case she became confused. She died two weeks later. The hospice staff were there, but she never got the chance to say goodbye to her children.

Mrs W taught me that we cannot always get it right, no matter how hard we try. Over the next few months I began to think about legalised assisted dying not as an admission of defeat, but as an insurance policy – rarely used but not entirely out of reach. The more I thought about it, the less sense did the arguments against make to me.

Take the claim that legalising assisted dying would stop palliative care in its tracks. The British Society of Geriatricians suggests that, 'The focus would shift from providing the best palliative care, i.e. easing symptoms, to providing death on demand.' I simply do not accept this.

The reason that thousands of doctors and nurses keep working to relieve symptoms is that we see people suffer every day, and we desperately want to help. As long as there are patients who need them, we will keep looking for answers. Even in the Netherlands, where more people choose assisted dying than in any other country, the vast majority of people die a 'natural' death. Unless every patient in the country chooses to die by euthanasia, there will still be thousands who need palliative care.

The experience of Oregon gives the lie to the idea that palliative care and a vibrant hospice movement would be endangered. An official report on dying in the USA places Oregon in the top ten states in terms of quality of end-of-life care. Since assisted dying was made legal in Oregon palliative care has become a speciality in its own right, and over half of the people in Oregon are receiving hospice care when they die.

As for the accusation from Care Not Killing that assisted dying 'provides a bolthole for lazy doctors', that is, frankly, rubbish. Of course there are dodgy doctors out there – just as there are dodgy judges, dodgy policemen and fairly iffy parents. Of course we doctors get things wrong – all the time. When a journalist makes a mistake, the newspaper prints a retraction; when a doctor makes a mistake, a person may die. It's a huge responsibility, and one that we take very seriously. Doctors are human. We don't pretend to be perfect, but we do care passionately about our patients and we (almost) always do our best.

Of course there would need to be safeguards if assisted dying were made legal. It would be unthinkable if people felt pressured into ending their own lives because they felt they were a burden to others. It would do untold damage to my ability to build up trust with my patients if they suspected I might knock them off when they were too much like hard work. As Oregon has shown us, those safeguards are possible without a hint of the 'slippery slope'. We can – and we should – be able to develop a system which gives help to the tiny minority (and, perhaps, an 'insurance policy' to those who know it is there, even if they don't use it) without threatening the vast majority who want to die a 'natural' death.

I believe the Netherlands has gone too far. I cannot ever imagine helping someone to die if I wasn't absolutely sure that they themselves wanted it. I would never support euthanasia for children, even at their parents' most heartfelt request. I would want to have no part in assisted dying for anyone, child or adult, who was not capable of making a fully informed decision. That would include anyone suffering from dementia or in a coma.

Having said that, the legally binding Advanced Decision and Lasting Power of Attorney systems that we already have allow you to decide, when you are 'of sound mind and body', to refuse life-saving treatment if you become unable to make that decision for yourself in the future. At every stage, you have to make clear in writing that your decision stands 'even if life is at risk'. I have absolutely no doubt that if assisted dying were made legal in the UK, some of my patients would be equally determined to fight for a similar right to demand help in dying through the same legal system. Perhaps John's father, who so desperately wanted to die but who was not capable of making his own choices at the end, could have been spared.

Mrs W taught me that there are entirely valid reasons why so many people want death on their own terms. All through our medical training, we have the importance of patients' autonomy – their right to make decisions about their own bodies – drummed into us. If a patient wants to refuse a treatment they have an absolute right to do just that, even if they die as a result. Yet here we are refusing them that same autonomy over the most important question of all.

As Professor John Harris, a philosopher, put it, 'It is only by the exercise of autonomy that our lives become in any real sense our own. The ending of our lives determines life's final shape and meaning, both for ourselves and in the eyes of others. When we are denied control at the end of our lives, we are denied autonomy.'

When one man dies, one chapter is not torn out of the book, but translated into a better language; and every chapter must be so translated.

John Donne

15

Last Words

I was close to finishing this book when I had a phone call from my younger brother Rob. He told me he was dying, though that's not exactly how he put it. What he said was that he had finished writing his autobiography, had noticed a pain in his chest and had gone to see his doctor. The doctor had found a massive tumour on his lung. It turned out to be malignant. What Rob wanted me to say was that he was not dying, that he would be one of the few who, in the absurd tabloid language we use for this subject, would battle the cancer and emerge victorious. So that's more or less what I told him, even though I did not believe it and neither did he. It's what you do in those circumstances, isn't it? Actually, I'm really not sure any longer that it is, but I'll come back to that. Rob – who had followed me into journalism and become the leading sports broadcaster in Wales – asked me if I would have a look at something he had written a few hours after his doctor delivered the news. And it really was a few hours; he wrote it while he was trying to get hold of me and his wife Julie. This is it:

You shouldn't be reading this about me!

Hell, I shouldn't be writing this about me!

You should be reading this about somebody else and I should be writing this about somebody else. Except I'm not. It is about me. There's an awful lot of 'me's there, but I'm rather afraid this is a subject where 'I', 'me' and 'my' are going to dominate, because it's not happening to somebody else. It's going to affect lots more – my wife, my three kids, even my cats who seem remarkably aware of my change of mood in the last three hours – but the bottom line is that it's me who's got to face this thing. This thing called 'death'. There, I've said it. It's only been three hours, and already I'm coming to terms with my own mortality.

Maybe I've been coming to terms with it for a bit longer than that – ever since my doctor, Trevor, who also doubles up as a friend, said I could probably do with an X-ray to sort out some pains I was getting in my chest and shoulder. I put it down to writing this book, crouched over a laptop on the kitchen table. Bad posture, got to be. Nothing to worry about. He sort of agreed – he might even be able to write it up in a medical journal – but, just to be on the safe side …

I made the appointment with the hospital. 'Next week?' asked the girl on reception. 'Bit difficult … how about the week after?' She looked at her appointments. 'It's a Bank Holiday on the Monday. How about Tuesday the 27th?' We had a deal. But what if I'd said I couldn't make it on the 27th? What if I had a prearranged filling at the dentist's or just didn't fancy getting up early after a Bank-Holiday night out? Then, I wouldn't be feeling like this now. I'd be in that blissful state of ignorance. I'd still be blaming bad posture, swallowing the odd anti-inflammatory and worrying about the credit crunch and the price of fuel. But no, I'd said I'd go on the 27th and I did.

It's funny how fate jumps in front of you, pulls a funny face and runs off cackling when you're facing up to inner fears. I was having an innocent Sunday evening pint with the papers at the pub after Manchester United's Champions League win against Chelsea a few days earlier. I was tempted to skip the match report – I'd wanted Chelsea to win after all – but I'd paid for the *Sunday Times* and I was going to read it.

There was a passage that leapt out at me, a poignant memory from Alex Ferguson about his dad:

'There are too many examples of people who retire and are in their box soon after. Because you are taking away the very thing that makes you alive, that keeps you alive. I remember my dad had his sixty-fifth birthday and the Fairfields shipyard gave him a dinner in Glasgow with four hundred people there. It was a big night for my dad. I was in Aberdeen and came down for it on a Friday. The next week my mother phoned and said, "Your dad's going in for an X-ray, he has pains in the chest." I said, "It'll be emotion." Well, it was cancer. A week, one week.'

Thanks, Sir Alex. Just what I wanted to hear. I've just retired, I've got pains in my chest and I'm going for an X-ray. That's all I need to read. But then a big furry creature called 'Rationalisation' appears and puts his arm around me. 'C'mon, Bob,' he purrs. 'How many people have an X-ray for pains in the chest and are soaking up the sun in St Tropez as we speak? Well, yeah, OK, not many, but that's down to the exchange rate of the pound against the euro rather than the fact that they've ended up in their box. Anyway, old Fergie was writing about the mid-eighties. Think how treatment has progressed since then!'

'You're right, Big R,' I reasoned and turned over to read the headline: 'The Exodus Begins'. The *Sunday Times* was talking about Avram Grant leaving Chelsea. For a moment I thought they might be on about me!

The X-rays were deceptively mundane. 'George Robert Humphrys?' a nurse calls out. It helps having an abbreviation as your work name. It saves the embarrassment of having the old ladies in their cardigans turning to their husbands and saying, 'Ooh look ... it's him off the telly. Does the sport or something!' A couple of quick clicks, 'Put your shirt back on' – a merciful release for the woman pressing the button – a slightly apprehensive jest about 'Got a good picture?' and it's time to go home. 'Your doctor should have the results in a week ... but ring before you go. They might not have turned up by then.'

That wasn't so bad, then. Even if the local evening paper does chip in with a story about a woman raising money for Velindre, Wales's specialist cancer treatment centre. Her husband was telling the story – about her organising a ball to raise funds for the hospital. The sting in the tail? She herself was diagnosed with lung cancer and died five weeks later, before the ball could be held. Jeez, not good, I thought. Five weeks? That's barely the time it takes to work out one of Garth Crooks's interminable post-match questions. Where's my old pal 'Rationalisation' when you need him?

I didn't have to ring the doctor before I went to see him for the results. He came to me. It was about four hours ago. I'd just had a phone call from my wife about getting the road tax done for our daughter's car, followed by another more tetchy one as she rang again two minutes later for more details from our bank card. 'Couldn't you have asked that five minutes ago?' I muttered irritably. It was probably the last time in my life I'm going to be annoyed about minutiae.

Two minutes later the doorbell was sounding. I'd bought the ridiculous chiming set of ring tones to annoy Julie a few years ago, so it could have been the 'Happy Birthday' tune or maybe 'Au clair de la lune'. I didn't notice. I was more concerned about the figure just about discernible through the stained glass. It was Trevor. This was not good.

I guessed there was something wrong. He knew there was something wrong. Somehow small talk about the weather seemed out of place.

'I don't know how to say this, Bob.' I was tempted to point out that if he didn't know how to do it, perhaps he shouldn't try, but I didn't. The time for being a smart arse had gone. 'You've got a mass on your lung ... it's malignant.'

Aah, I was right, this was not good. Not good at all. What are you meant to say? How about, 'I watched an episode of *House* a couple of weeks ago, Trev. Guy on there was diagnosed with lung cancer and it turned out they were wrong. He sued them for millions. Better make sure you're right on this one, boy!' Somehow, that didn't strike the right tone either. I rather think that if he rings the doorbell now and says, 'Sorry, mate, bad batch of film ... bit of a mistake, there's nothing wrong with the X-ray at all. Carry on as normal', I'd waltz him round the room and open a bottle of my 1983 St Emilion Grand Cru rather than get on the phone to Lawyers-for-you.

There was a bit of a chat about CT scans and discovering whether it was secondary or primary, but I thought this was no time to discuss schools. It did, though, seem rather unjust. I'd had one puff of a cigarette in my life when I was ten, and had spent all of the following day throwing up. Punishment enough, it seemed, but no! Lung cancer was meant to affect those who smoked cigarettes next to me in pubs all my adult life. Maybe there was a clue there. I'd always been in favour of the smoking ban in pubs. It's just a pity it was all a little late.

'I think I'd probably prefer to be alone, Trev.' What a dreadful line, I might have said on any other occasion, totally over the top, much too melodramatic, and then I realised it was me saying it. Did I want him to go? I suppose I had to tell my wife. She didn't answer her phone, probably pissed off with my earlier irritability. I tried my brother. The fastest, least personal answerphone message in the world told me to leave a message and get off. I did. I thought that possibly this –

'Hi, John. Maybe – nope, probably – dying. Talk later. Cheers' – was a bit terse, even for his busy world.

I noticed my mobile phone was on the blink. Shit, this was definitely not my day! At least – unlike my wife and brother – Vodafone answered eventually. The girl at the end of the line, who might or might not have been recording my call for training purposes, sounded remarkably chipper. 'Whoa, my lovely,' I was tempted to say in my most patronising way, 'I want none of this bonhomie. I'll have you know I've just received news that I could be about to shuffle off the old mortal coil. I could soon be an ex-person.'

I didn't, of course. I just listened as she told me the nearest store to take the Nokia N95 to. I wondered if they could fix malignant masses on the lung too.

The world outside the front door seemed awfully normal. The car was just as I had left it last night. A weird thought came into my mind about how life – like history – could now be divided into two: BC and AD ... 'Before Confirmation' and 'After Diagnosis'. BC was everything up to an hour ago; AD is everything since. They're very different places. AD – and I've only been here five or so hours now – has me looking at the woman pushing the shopping trolley or the workman shovelling the cafeteria lunch into his mouth and thinking, 'So what's the biggest problem in your life, eh? A pint of milk being the price of a long weekend in Paris, the fact your darts team lost last night? Pah, luxury, a mere bagatelle ... I can beat yah hollow.'

There will need to be readjustments. I bumped into an acquaintance as I went to fill a prescription in the local chemist – I suspect there'll be a lot of that in the future – and there was the usual, means-nothing greetings: 'Hi, Dickie ... all right?' 'Yeah, Bob ... you?' 'Fine.' 'Fine!' I'm telling him I'm *fine*! I'm not fine at all. I'm walking and I'm talking, but inside I'm feeling like one of those characters shuffling along in *Night of the Living Dead*. 'I'm not one of you any more, Dickie ... the pod has hatched inside me!'

On the television the hammer still comes down on antiques that people didn't really want to sell in the first place, would-be homebuyers look at properties that would have been 30 per cent cheaper if they'd waited until now, and C-list celebrities salivate over what a TV chef can do with a chicken leg and a bunch of carrots. It's all so familiar yet so alien. And outside the rain still comes down. It reminds me of a conversation I had with a friend when I was about twelve. It was chucking it down and we were talking for some reason about funerals. 'I want it to be raining really hard when it's mine,' I said. 'That way everyone will be miserable with me!' There was an obvious flaw in the argument of the twelve-year-old me, but I know how he felt. I feel like that now.

So what does the future hold six hours AD? Do I go to the pub and smile and joke and pretend everything's all right? Do I Google 'malignant masses on the lung' and scare myself shitless? Do I email the BBC's Pensions Department and say, 'You know I ticked that box saying I didn't want to take an enhanced pension until I was sixty-five? Is it too late to change my mind?'

I've told my wife now, but John's answerphone is still on. My son Jamie is doing his GCSEs. Would knowing affect his chances in the exams? Should I tell my daughter Claire, the vet, who texted me this morning to ask the results of my tests? And what about Emma, who's just finished her university finals? She should be enjoying herself, not thinking about me.

There's much to ponder. Will I sleep tonight? That prescription might help ... it was for Temazepam. And will there be much pain? I don't think I'm keen on pain. It has to be said, I'm scared ...

Rob was right to be scared. Seven weeks after Trevor had knocked on his door to tell him he had a tumour, he was dead. I grieve for him. What a stupidly obvious thing to write. Of course I grieve for him. He was my younger brother – the little boy who had tormented me when I was a young teenager as only little boys can and then, when we'd both grown up a bit, had become my best friend. His death was a savage blow to his wife Julie, to his three children, to his many friends and to me.

As I write Rob's face looks up at me from the cover of his brilliant autobiography, which was published a few weeks after his funeral. There is a half smile, a quizzical expression which nicely captures his approach to life – sometimes puzzled but mostly amused. I imagine, as I look at it, that there is a hint of reproach in it too. Of course that's fanciful – the photograph was taken long before the fatal diagnosis, when he was living life to the full – but it doesn't alter the fact that I feel I let him down when he most needed me. Just as I feel I let down my father and my former wife.

Psychiatrists tell us that guilt is a common component of the grief we feel when someone who was very close to us dies. We dredge up all the things we did and said over the years that we later came to regret. We hate ourselves for having said things we should not have said and for having left unspoken so many things we should have said – especially in those final days. We are desperate to make amends when it is too late – even if there was never really anything to make amends for. Common sense dictates that there has never been a relationship between two people – however much they may have loved each other – in which it has been all sweetness and light, but common sense goes out of the window in those dark days when grief is at its most intense and the pain is most real. The guilt may be entirely irrational, but grief and reason are not natural bedfellows.

That has always been the case and I suppose it always will be, but in other ways, as our approach to death has changed over the decades, so has our approach to grief. We have largely lost the quiet, private expression of grief for those we mourn which was expressed perfectly by Wilfred Owen in his 'Anthem for Doomed Youth': 'And each slow dusk, a drawing down of blinds.' Owen was writing about another era, when tears were shed in private and dignity and reserve were displayed in public. Now it seems to have gone into reverse – perhaps because of the insatiable demands of the television cameras. Instead we have the banality of the 'How do you feel about the death of your child?' interview; the bathetic spectacle of flowers laid publicly at the spot where someone died in an accident; the collective hysteria over the death of someone we have met only in the columns of newspapers or on our television screens. When Princess Diana died it was not real grief we witnessed during that awful week of national mourning. It was mass emoting – as unhealthy and unreal as it was synthetic and orchestrated.

I was at a concert in London's Albert Hall five days after Diana's terrible accident. The main piece was to be a Mozart piano concerto. Instead, the conductor announced that it was being replaced – as a mark of respect for the dead Princess – by a requiem. Oh, and we were solemnly instructed not to applaud at the end of it. You could sense many in the audience shuffling, irritated by the change of programme and embarrassed by the whole thing, but nobody said anything. They were scared of causing offence. There is a kind of grief fascism that operates on those occasions and I find it slightly frightening. Real grief is not paraded. It is not worn like a badge. It is private.

And something else has changed. When death was a natural part of life, grief was a natural part of living. Now there is a tendency to treat it as an unwelcome affliction, or the symptom of an illness which must be treated. When a child dies the other children in the school may be offered counselling, which has always struck me as both odd and potentially damaging. Left to their own devices, most children have an extraordinary ability to come to terms with tragedy. They have a way of compartmentalising, putting sad events into context, recognising that some things happen which they can do nothing about, and then getting on with their lives. Obviously there are exceptions. If their own lives are dramatically affected by the death of a parent or a sibling, that's quite different and they may well need help, but turning private grief counselling into a public industry is not the way to do it.

In this book Sarah and I have tried to explore what it is that constitutes a good death. The attitude of modern society to death has changed because our attitude to life has changed. A century ago we knew that death was never far away and we were prepared for it. Today the opposite is true. Now our minds seem unprepared for what our bodies are doing. I am not suggesting that there should be a morbid preoccupation with death. Quite the contrary. As someone who had a new baby at an age when my grandfather would have been contemplating the end of his life I can only wonder at my good fortune. For me life did not end at sixty: a new life began. And there are many, many more like me. For that we should give thanks. God knows, I do.

Our ancestors would have envied us our longevity, but could not have anticipated the pain it has brought to some. My father lived a much longer life than most people born before the First World War and, like so many of them, became as much a victim as a beneficiary of his extra years. Medical advances meant we could keep him alive and so that is what we did – in spite of his own wishes – and the result was that his final descent into senility cast a shadow over his life. His misery was compounded by his sense that he had lost control over his life and his death. His wishes were disregarded.

Rob was still in his fifties, with everything to live for, and his illness – unlike our father's – was swift and deadly. But there was one grim comparison to be made. Rob, too, felt he had lost control. His final weeks were blighted by the sense that others were making decisions for him. I had encouraged him to believe that he could beat the cancer when I should have been encouraging him to accept what we all knew was inevitable. He hated and feared what was happening to him: the ultimate loss of control and dignity. He hated it so much that he turned his face to the wall. For one dreadful period towards the end he refused to see anyone but his wife, who had to assume the role not only of comforter but also of doctor and nurse. He would allow no one else into his room.

When Julie told him I was driving down to Cardiff, he told her he did not want to see me. I got in the car anyway. I was halfway down the M4 when he phoned and – in a voice I barely recognised – told me to turn back. I refused. When I walked into his bedroom he told me to leave. Again I refused.

Eventually he relented and we spent the rest of the day talking.

It was a good conversation, but I did not say all the things I now wish I had said, and it was to be our last. He told me that what he wanted above all else was for everyone to leave him alone. Julie did everything humanly possible to help him through those final days, but even she could not give him the only thing he wanted. He wanted to be in control of his own death just as he had been in control of his own life until the moment the cancer struck.

The day after I returned to London Rob was rushed into hospital because his lungs were filling with fluid. When I got there he was drifting in and out of consciousness. His doctor assured Julie and me that he would do nothing to try to keep him alive and he was true to his word; but it was more than twenty-four hours after Rob was admitted before the last, shuddering breath left his body.

I wish his final few days had been different. When I held his hand in his bedroom and we had our last real conversation and he told me what he feared, I wish I had been able to say to him: 'You are in control. We both know you are dying. It is for you and nobody else to decide how and when your life comes to its end. If you want help to die, we will give you that help.'

But I could not – any more than I could help my father to die – and I shall never forgive myself for that. I let them down. I believe that the dying have at least the same rights as the living: above all, the right to make their own decisions, to take control of the end of their lives in the way they wish. Anything less is a form of betrayal.